EMF off!

A call to consciousness

in our misguidedly microwaved world

by Olga Sheean

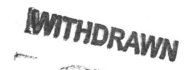

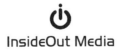

InsideOut Media

A note on the resources and references included in this book

Since everything in our world is changing so rapidly, information in a book can quickly become obsolete. While website links are printed in this book, readers are advised to go to https://emfoff.com/resources for a complete list of references by chapter, as well as other resources that become available over time. Further reading can be found at https://emfoff.com/blog.

Praise for *EMF off!*

"Olga Sheean's book is a wake-up call for us all. Beautifully written, it describes her own severe health effects from EMFs, as well as the science on electromagnetic radiation, while providing hope and inspiration for creating a better world. May everyone who cares about health, the environment and our common future on this planet read this book and become part of the growing web of consciousness. *Be the change you want to see in the world.*"

—*Mona Nilsson, journalist, founder/chair of Swedish Radiation Protection Foundation, and author of* Health Risks of Wireless Technology

"A call to consciousness on many levels, *EMF off!* is informative, smart, sad and funny all at once. The touching afterword, written by Olga's husband Lewis, will be helpful to other couples facing similar challenges. A must-read for a holistic view of the global effects of EMF in this technological age."

—*Jolie Jones, artist, author, environmental activist, producer (Jolietalks.com)*

"This is an important book from someone with wide experience and a unique background. Olga shares her deep insights into both the personal devastation caused by man-made EMF energy and the vested interests that have hindered public health action to prevent such harm. Her analysis of the wireless dangers that society faces is balanced by empowering solutions made possible by scientific advances."

—*Michael Bevington, Chair of Electrosensitivity UK (es-uk.info) and author of* Electromagnetic Sensitivity and Electromagnetic Hypersensitivity—a summary

"Powerful, joyous, painful, witty, illuminating and memorable, this book is a rich montage by a masterful writer, with a story that traverses many landscapes. As microwave radiation permeates every aspect of her life, Olga becomes a silent observer in a world where she can no longer fully engage. '*Yet, due to my isolation and emptiness, I am gaining insights that I might not otherwise have gained.*' Armed with knowledge, an irrepressible spirit and an irreverent sense of humour, Olga travels a journey of self-discovery and empowerment, revealing many of the ingredients essential to our well-being and the survival of our planet. Highly recommended to anyone seeking betterment, this book will find a home in your heart."

—*Denise Rowland, human rights activist, writer and performer*

"Olga Sheean takes us on an intimate personal journey. Along the way, she challenges us to cultivate our deeper truth, reconnect and choose love. Our relationship with technology is like nothing our society has ever faced, and only we can cure our own addiction. I'm so thankful for this book."

—*Theodora Scarato, MSW, Executive Director, Environmental Health Trust*
(https://ehtrust.org/)

"Sheean's words help to water the over-digitised desert—both inner and outer—into which humanity, steeped in wireless-product marketing, is perceptibly heading with gathering speed. Whatever your current understanding of this field, I encourage you to read this book with an open mind and, through it, recover that pearl-beyond-price, the Precautionary Principle, and the inner strength to serve it."

—*Lynne Wycherley, environmentalist, writer and poet*

"On her odyssey back to health, Olga Sheean treads the little known but increasingly common pathway of illnesses caused by chemical and electrical sensitivity. Her story is one that everyone needs to hear as these devastating illnesses pervade our increasingly contaminated world.

"This book emphasizes how many of the precursors to electrical and chemical problems can be prevented, outlining what we have learned about EMF sensitivity over the last 40 years, and reminding us that the body runs on electricity, as evidenced by EKG, EEG and EMG.

"Radiation from WiFi, smart meters, cellular phones, computers and TVs can have a serious impact on the body, causing it to malfunction in ways that cannot be resolved with medication. We should all use this information as a preventative tool for our own long-term well-being."

—*Dr William Rea, MD, Founder/Director, Environmental Health Center–Dallas*

"Rare is the storyteller who weaves a tapestry of truth, science, environmental alerts, quantum physics and spirituality, laced with sheer determination and humor. Sheean pulls no punches in outlining the health impacts to humans, animals and planet from electromagnetic fields, along with empowering solutions for dealing with this invisible force, while protecting ourselves and our loved ones. A must-read, if ever there was one!"

—*Christine S. Zipps, health rights advocate, nutritionist and nature photographer*

"Current research is revealing that, within just five generations of low-level microwave irradiation, exposed species—from soil microorganisms to mammalian vertebrates and all plant life in between—could become extinct. Confronting what is arguably the most powerful opposing force on this planet, this book is an inspiration for those who wish to leave our world fit for all forms of life."

—*Barrie Trower, research physicist and specialist in microwave radiation*

"Drawing on traumatic personal experience and extensive research, Olga Sheean documents the pervasive impact of electromagnetic radiation on our lives, spelling out the dangers and proposing countermeasures and solutions. The use of metaphors and figures of speech enhances her writing and makes the message more compelling—*a vote of confidence in ourselves; a tsunami of consciousness; global disconnectedness*. Think: *elevating your frequencies.*

"As the fourth industrial revolution inexorably overwhelms the environment, one fears that matters will get worse before they get better, with the domestication of radiation through the Internet of Things. As a disability activist, I realize that sensitivity to electromagnetic radiation has yet to be recognized as the disabling condition that it is. I encourage all to read, learn, and join us in activism."

—*Dr William Rowland, author of* Nothing About Us Without Us: Inside the Disability Rights Movement of South Africa, *award-winning activist, Honorary President of Disabled People of South Africa (DPSA), and Chair of the 2009 UN Assembly, launching the Convention for the Rights of People with Disabilities*

"Anyone who has experienced electromagnetic hypersensitivity (EHS) will relate to this informative book. The delightful writing style will take you on a rollercoaster ride through the world of those affected by electrosmog pollution, which permeates all corners of modern society.

"Those with EHS fall through the cracks of our medical system, as the majority of physicians remain uninformed about this emerging health crisis, despite the global outcry from hundreds of EMF scientists and physicians against the expansion of electromagnetic radiation.

"We consider ourselves privileged to have become friends with Olga and Lewis, on our own journey through the life-altering effects of this serious public health issue, while governments remain stuck in bureaucratic paralysis, just as they were with asbestos, tobacco etc, not long ago."

—*Benita & Marcus Schluschen*

Dedication

This book is dedicated to the many independent scientists,
researchers, doctors, educators and activists who work tirelessly
to promote awareness of the adverse biological effects of
manmade electromagnetic radiation in our environment.
We owe them our profound gratitude for dedicating their time,
knowledge and expertise towards restoring
a healthy balance in our world.

Contents

PART 3: UNCOVERING THE DEEPER TRUTH

PART 4: THE CALL TO CONSCIOUSNESS

Acronyms and terms used in the text

Electro-sensitivity: More commonly referred to in the medical literature as electromagnetic hypersensitivity (EHS), electro-sensitivity is a sensitivity to electromagnetic fields, which results in multiple biological effects. The term is often used interchangeably with microwave sickness; however, the latter does not reflect the fact that many individuals are also sensitive to the extremely low frequencies (ELFs) that are not in the RF/microwave range.

EMF: An electromagnetic field (sometimes called an EM field) is the space in which an electrical charge can be detected. It is generated when charged particles, such as electrons, are accelerated. All electrically charged particles are surrounded by electric fields. Charged particles in motion produce magnetic fields. When the velocity of a charged particle changes, an electromagnetic field is produced.

EMR: In physics, electromagnetic radiation refers to the waves of the electromagnetic field, propagating through space-time, carrying electromagnetic radiant energy. This form of radiation includes visible light, radio waves, gamma rays and x-rays, in which electric and magnetic fields vary simultaneously.

Microwave radiation: Microwave radiation is a form of electromagnetic radiation between radio waves and infrared waves on the electromagnetic spectrum, with frequencies of between 300MHz and 300GHz and wavelengths of between 1 metre and 1 millimetre.

1

Microwave sickness: A condition of impaired health, reported especially in the Russian medical literature, that is characterized by headaches, anxiety, sleep disturbances, fatigue, difficulty concentrating, and changes in the cardiovascular and central nervous systems, caused by prolonged exposure to low-intensity microwave radiation.[1]

Non-ionizing radiation: Non-ionizing radiation includes visible, infra-red and ultraviolet light; microwaves; radio waves; and radio-frequency energy from cell phones.

Neuroplasticity: Neuroplasticity refers to the brain's ability to change its own structure and functioning in response to mental activities and emotional focus.

Quantum physics: Quantum physics is the science that explains the properties of solids, atoms, nuclei, sub-nuclear particles and light. In order for us to understand these natural phenomena, quantum principles have required fundamental changes in how humans view nature. The quantum world is a world of infinite possibilities, with consciousness playing a key role in what ultimately becomes matter. And matter (whether in the form of our bodies or the universe itself) is far less dense than we imagine, made up of space more than anything else.

Radio-frequency radiation: Radio-frequency (RF) electromagnetic radiation is the transfer of energy by radio waves. It lies in the frequency range between 3kHz and 300GHz.

Radiowave sickness: Another term for microwave sickness.

Universal intelligence: Universal intelligence is often described as divine guidance, answered prayers, miracles or anything that helps us accomplish what may seem impossible in light of the physical limitations in our physical world. It is the unified field of universal energy of which we are all an integral part and through which we are all interconnected. Although beyond the level of our normal waking consciousness, it is fully accessible to us.

WiFi radiation: Radio-frequency microwave radiation produced by WiFi routers and wireless devices.

Foreword

This book tells a poignant, deeply personal story that will resonate with many of us and serve as a warning to everyone else. Punctuated with wry humour and many revelations, it is a story that evolves—from a purely personal perspective to one of planetary relevance. On her journey through electromagnetic hypersensitivity (EHS), from the initial disturbing, inexplicable symptoms, to the development of a brain tumour and beyond, Olga Sheean learned first-hand the adverse effects of microwave radiation and its impact on every aspect of her life. But she did not stop there.

Many people will relate to her challenges of consulting doctors who do not understand the condition, and of having to figure out solutions for herself. Olga shares the science of how man-made electromagnetic radiation affects all forms of life, as well as the frustration of presenting the truth to the establishment ...and being met with flat denial. For her, this denial prompted a deeper exploration of the factors that have taken us to the brink of our tolerance—in our bodies and in our environment—and a deeper understanding of what it all represents.

Our environment has changed dramatically over the last 150 years, since the invention of AC (alternating current) electricity. We are now exposed to levels of electromagnetic and radio-frequency fields billions of times greater than the background levels that our biology was designed for. These fields affect our biology in both thermal and non-thermal ways.

Research in Russia from the 1930s onwards has recognized this and, in the Western world, military and industrial research in the 1950s and 1960s focused on exploiting these effects in the development of microwave weapons ...and found evidence of biological effects from non-thermal electromagnetic fields. Despite these non-thermal effects, European and North American safety limits for electromagnetic radiation from wireless technologies are inexplicably set for thermal effects only—in other words, only when a heating effect is considered to occur.

The huge profits generated by the telecommunications industry may explain why non-thermal effects are being discounted and ignored. If the issue of non-thermal effects is raised, authorities can then pretend that they are irrelevant, and engineers have the widest possible latitude to exploit areas of the electromagnetic spectrum, and to 'smog' our environment while avoiding any responsibility or legal liability.

Human progress over the last millennium has seen revolutions in literacy, agriculture, industry, transport, power generation and communications. The latest revolution—that of information technology—has transformed our world faster and more profoundly than any other in our history. In all of these revolutions, society derives new opportunities and abilities, as well as a greater potential for the expression of human consciousness.

However, progress always brings problems as well as opportunities, and safety always lags behind technological advances …with the dangers initially hidden. Society always takes time to change its thinking about any controversial issue, progressing from outright denial to gradual acceptance and recognition: *there isn't a problem; there are a few mad people who say there's a problem; there's a very small problem; we have a problem, but it's completely under control;* and, finally, *oh my God, we have a problem!*

This is particularly true when dealing with wireless technology and mobile connectivity because they are so useful and seductive. While many technological advances have helped us immeasurably, society is having a difficult time coming to terms with the fact that its addiction to wireless devices and connectivity carries significant risks and harms—not just in terms of symptoms, but also at deeper biological levels and in our environment. The addiction to devices among children is particularly worrying, and the escalating incidence of disease is also a serious concern. The tragedy lies in the mistaken presumption of no harm.

Increasing numbers of people are connecting their symptoms of poor sleep, fatigue, dizziness, cognitive impairment, headaches, tingling, palpitations and pains (all of which I have observed in my patients) with exposure to radio-frequency/microwave fields—and all experience relief when they remove themselves from the fields. This is not surprising, since human beings are electromagnetic. Our cells function and communicate using electricity at minute voltages and power ratings, and also using biophotons. Bodies sense tiny electromagnetic fields and convert them into physical and chemical reactions—for instance, the eyes can sense a single photon, the ears a billionth of a watt.

The tragedy lies in the mistaken presumption of no harm.

Symptoms alert us to disharmony in the mind-body-spirit, prompting us to recognize problems and avert greater harm. This book offers empowering approaches to resolving all aspects of health—reducing exposure to electromagnetic pollution, using nutrition and physical and emotional nourishment, resolving negative emotions, understanding the impact of our emotional dysfunction, and (most challenging for a society entrained by materialism and devices) evolving our level of consciousness.

When we disconnect the human head (our clever intellect) from the human heart (compassion), we reap untold problems. If we reconnect head and heart, calm the chattering mind, and pay attention to what our soul is telling us through our heart, perhaps we can individually and collectively forge a promising future. If we demand that engineers, industry and governments incorporate respect for all forms of life into our modern technologies, they will rise to the challenge. When guided by such wisdom and by a global demand for healthier alternatives, society will always find ingenious solutions.

Whatever vision we hold for our world, it must be based on the values of respect and compassion for all forms of life. These values resonate with every one of us, and they are in tune with the constructive power of consciousness, which modern physicists and philosophers tell us underpins the very existence of the universe.

Composed of hardware (our body) and software (our soul), we are individual vehicles for consciousness. We are all here on a journey of learning in life, exploring the experience of consciousness in matter. We are spiritual beings having a physical experience, evolving and developing, manipulating our environment, and learning about relationships with others and with our environment. We can act wisely ...or not. Many live life as a passive experience, rather than a journey of personal development as a being and soul. If the latter is appreciated, then people take responsibility, understand the drama triangle of victim, rescuer and persecutor, and start to use the rules and tools of personal development proactively.

When guided by wisdom and a global demand for healthier alternatives, society will always find ingenious solutions.

The need for us to reconnect with our hearts and our spiritual selves is one of the key messages in this book. If we disregard our spirituality, we fill this gap with (external) material possessions, and an exploration of the physical and technological world, while neglecting our (internal) soul's maturity. Society fails to appreciate that, as agents of consciousness, we each have untold power and ability to make a difference, in accordance with how much we follow our soul's guidance, and how much we develop our character and qualities, such as compassion. Focusing on the physical world, and using chemistry to explore biology and medicine, without integrating modern physics, has given us an incomplete understanding of human bodies and beings. When we ignore the development of our souls, we develop imbalances of mind-body-spirit and become unwell, with the body communicating with us in many of the ways described in these pages.

In this book, Olga acts as a courageous messenger for all of society, urging us to explore the deeper implications of our technologically driven lifestyles, to regain our autonomy, to take an empowered approach to resolving the current EMF crisis, and to elevate our consciousness to create a healthier world with happier people. The depletion of our environment and the rapid global rise in health problems confirm the urgent need for us to regain control over our physical, emotional, nutritional, environmental and spiritual well-being.

With wisdom and relevance for every one of us, whether symptomatic of EHS or not, this book explains why EMFs are such a devastating environmental pollutant—which, if not addressed, will decimate our pollinators, compromise our fertility and DNA, and bring the human race to a very precarious place. It inspires us to acknowledge the responsibility we have to ourselves, to others, and to the whole of consciousness.

—Dr Andrew Tresidder, MBBS, Cert. Med. Ed.,
Physician Health Educator, Trustee of ES-UK, former Family Physician

Introduction

There is a disturbing phenomenon sweeping the planet. Beneath the feeding frenzy surrounding the wireless technologies that have transformed the pace and nature of our lives, there's a dark underbelly of dysfunction. On the surface, an epidemic is emerging, with millions of people being adversely affected by the rapidly proliferating electromagnetic radiation in our environment (including the microwave radiation from WiFi, cell towers, cell/cordless phones and other wireless devices).

> **"Ten percent of the population is already suffering the damaging effects of 4G and WiFi radiation, yet doctors and scientists are failing to recognize this because of the sheer diversity of illnesses it's causing."**
>
> —Prof. Trevor Marshall, Director,
> Autoimmunity Research Foundation, California

The now unavoidable over-exposure to electromagnetic fields (EMFs) is resulting in an explosion of physical conditions, cancers and neurological disorders, including electromagnetic hypersensitivity (EHS), often referred to as electro-sensitivity or microwave sickness.[2] Even though this is arguably the largest and most rapidly growing epidemic in our history, and countless scientific studies confirm the harmful biological effects of EMFs,[3] it is being largely ignored by governments. Now heavily influenced by—and beholden to—the massive wireless telecommunications industry, governments are refusing to openly acknowledge the proven dangers. But there's another aspect to their denial, and understanding it may prove crucial to our survival.

The invasive irradiation of our global environment is one of the inevitable outcomes of the way we, as a society, have been living our lives—focusing on technology at the expense of our well-being, depleting our natural resources, and failing to make healthy choices, in harmony with nature.

We are being pushed to correct this imbalance—firstly, within ourselves, by healing our bodies and addressing the emotional dysfunction that drives our behaviour; and, secondly, in our world, by reclaiming the autonomy and personal responsibility we have surrendered to governments, industry and those exploiting our environment. Having abdicated responsibility for key aspects of our existence, many of us are now losing control over our bodies as well as our environments—and never has the inextricable connection between the two been more alarmingly clear.

It's our playground; it's our source of food; it's our home. It is our life-support system. But our environment is also a sounding board for our growth. It's where we get to test our limits, our level of social responsibility, our creativity and our humanity. The current state of our environment is not just a passive reflection of how we operate or what we've done to ourselves; it's also an active push to empowerment.

With the advent of wireless radiation, we're losing control over the very atmosphere that sustains us, with many of us being pushed to the brink of our tolerance. It's a test of our conviction in our right to exist. We can document the damage, but this is not about berating ourselves for what we have done wrong; it's about understanding that our circumstances and our environment hold the clues for our recovery. They are telling us what is missing in our lives and what we need to do to regain a healthy balance and to thrive.

How bad do things have to get before we take assertive action? And what is our environment reflecting back to us about ourselves that we can use to regain our essential connection and humanity?

When push comes to shovel (the one that digs your grave)

Electro-sensitivity may well be a last desperate cry for a return to a world of meaningful connection, respect, balance and healthy self-acceptance. Emotional/physical sensitivity can be a life-saving faculty, alerting us to danger, and to deny its validity is to deny our very humanness. It should not surprise us that so many are sensitive to the electromagnetic fields in our highly irradiated environment and that they become sick or functionally impaired. Those affected can end up losing an entire lifetime of accumulated assets, expertise, community, social life, home and professional advancement. When people are deprived of life's commodities, backed into a corner of lonely isolation, and stripped of all the external distractions, they can lose their identity and sense of belonging. Many are so incapacitated that they cannot function normally, engage productively in society or access the goods or services they need to live a normal, healthy, productive life.

Yet challenging governments and service-providers and holding them accountable is not working. Governments, as well as non-governmental health authorities such as the International EMF Project of the World Health Organization (WHO), are denying that there is a problem, that microwave radiation is dangerous, and even that electro-sensitivity exists. After decades of us not holding ourselves or them accountable for what's happening to our planet, they see no reason to make themselves accountable to us now.

Many electro-sensitive individuals are being challenged to start again from scratch, using the power of their minds to find the strength and resilience to move forward. With a blank slate, they have an opportunity to return to first principles and to mindfully construct their own reality, reconnecting with their own innate powers of creativity and innovation and with the restorative powers of nature.

Saying 'NO' to technological addiction

Our obsession with being online has created a frenzy of non-stop connectivity that disrupts sleep, fragments families, undermines personal relationships, disregards personal boundaries, creates addictions and disease, promotes neediness and self-loathing, and prevents us from ever truly being at peace or connecting with our deeper selves in the pursuit of what matters most. An addiction that's "harder to kick than drugs",[4] according to Dr Nicholas Kardaras, author of *Glow Kids*, 'digital heroin' is arguably the most pervasive and destructive recreational 'drug' in society. Our increasingly wireless lifestyle is also undermining our natural environment faster than anything else in our history, affecting plant and animal life, as well as crops and the bees and other pollinators upon which much of our food supply depends.

We can choose to evolve in healthy, sustainable ways. In doing what's healthy and best for our bodies and minds, we automatically do what's best for our environment. Addressing climate change, adopting sustainability policies, levying carbon taxes—none of these things will change *us*, the perpetrators of the damage that prompts such desperate yet futile efforts.

Our bodies hold all the clues we need

Because electromagnetic radiation can affect all body systems, ongoing exposure can cause a progressive system shutdown. Nervous system disorders, disrupted sleep, impaired immune systems, depleted hormones, reproductive problems, neurological/cognitive disorders, premature aging and degeneration, chronic inflammation and high oxidative stress: with ongoing, excessive exposure, this radiation can affect us on all levels. For many of those affected, the world has become an inhospitable place where they no longer feel included, acknowledged, respected or accommodated.

This rejection has created despair and hopelessness for many electro-sensitive individuals. *If our governments, communities, colleagues, friends and family won't help us, what hope do we have?* Yet this situation represents the culmination of the dysfunction that has been ongoing and deepening for a very long time. For as long as we humans have been able to communicate, we have been telling each other stories about what we are worth, what's possible for us and what we must do to gain acceptance and survive. Many of us have been programmed to believe that circumstances are beyond our control, that we must defer to authority, that we must compromise to get what we want, that love and acceptance must be earned, that others determine our value, that we do not have the power to master our own lives/bodies, and that we do not deserve to have an easy, joyful, fulfilling life. As a result, the qualities of acceptance, compassion, respect, validation, support and spiritual connection, so essential to our well-being and personal evolution, have been progressively eroded, while we focus increasingly on performance, convenience, profit and technological prowess.

The higher calling hidden in our crises

A growing number of us are starting to realize that we are being pushed, at a deeper level, to declare a vote of confidence in ourselves, rather than passively deferring to governments or politicians. What can we do that does not require their permission? What choices can we make that will enable us to start healing ourselves and our environment? How can we regain control over our own lives?

Seen from the perspective of us having the power—and responsibility—to reclaim our autonomy over our bodies, lives and environment, the epidemic of electro-sensitivity serves a higher purpose: that of triggering a deeper realization of just how far we have strayed from our humanity, our autonomy and our purpose, and what we must do to reclaim them. Our challenges can become our strengths, once we understand what they represent. The rapidly spreading phenomenon of functional impairment[5] caused by our irradiated environment challenges us to start heading back to a healthy reverence for ourselves and for our planet.

If we cannot live in our toxic environment and if we are not being heard by the authorities/industries that are harming us, we must use the power of our minds and spirits, in co-creation with universal intelligence, to take back control of our own lives.

This book will help you to do that, whether you have been knowingly affected by EMFs or not. It is divided into four parts:

1. **The story of harm**
   This includes my personal story of how I have been affected by EMFs and what I have learned, in the process (with some rather quirky humour).

2. **Fighting for our lives**
   This section presents the science on electromagnetic fields (EMFs), a medical explanation of electro-sensitivity, what you can do to enhance your well-being and personal environment, and some of the legal and other measures I have taken to address the issue.

3. **Uncovering the deeper truth**

   I explore the deeper dynamics—what's driving our reactive, addictive, self-destructive behaviour, our lives and our realities, and how we can give ourselves what we have been missing.

4. **The call to consciousness**

   This section offers empowered solutions for reclaiming our health, our autonomy and our life, combined with a call to consciousness designed to put us back in touch with our phenomenal co-creative powers and a deeper understanding of what we are being called upon to do.

Although this book focuses on addressing the adverse effects of man-made EMFs in our environment, it is designed to bring all of you back 'online', activating those parts of you that have become disconnected. Many of the solutions provided here will also help with personal crises and problems, since empowering you has a positive impact on all aspects of your life. The book explains that EMFs represent just one doorway to healing, awareness and wholeness, and why we have focused on technological supremacy at the expense of our humanity, autonomy and spiritual connection. It also offers inspiration for living with the kind of conscious connectedness that generates more breakthroughs, love, magic and fulfillment than our wireless devices could ever do.

I hope it will ignite in you a fierce determination to become the powerful individual you are neurologically and spiritually designed to be, while reminding you of the infinite possibilities that unfold when we collaborate to create the world we want.

We are all in this together.

—Olga Sheean

Note to the reader:

This book is not anti-technology; it is pro-humanity, pro-sanity and pro-survival. Many people believe that WiFi is the only way to access the Internet, having never known anything else, or having forgotten that things used to be hard-wired, not so long ago. As a writer and online therapist, I find my computer invaluable, but it is safely hard-wired to our Internet modem, providing all the benefits of online access without any of the adverse effects of WiFi microwave radiation.

PART 1
THE STORY OF HARM

1 Life is good

Where does the blue begin? I'm sunbathing on the balcony, contemplating the infinite blue sky and listening to the waves crash onto the shore 100 metres away, while the countless dogs of Granja village continue their incessant symphony of manic barks in every key. The blue seems solid and endless, starting at some indefinable point that is forever beyond my reach ...like the horizon—today, a strong, clear line above the shimmering waves of the Atlantic, which are cresting frothily below the wooden boardwalk that stretches as far as the eye can see in both directions.

I like Granja—apart from all the barking dogs—and our modest rented villa on Portugal's west coast has become a haven of simplicity, far from the clamour of modern civilisation. It's only for a month, yet our time here seems elastic—sometimes slowing almost to a standstill and sometimes speeding up to the tempo of a geriatric jog. While I spend my days editing a weighty document for the United Nations, punctuated with frequent sanity-saving breaks on the balcony, languid meals made from our favourite Mediterranean foods, wines warmed in the hot sun on the windowsill, and skin-tingling walks along the sand-swept beach, Lewis works on his book—tap-tapping steadily on his keyboard in the other room, the sun streaming in behind him from the open window and the ocean breeze salting his mind with ideas. It's his first novel, yet it's flowing out of him effortlessly, chapter after chapter, with no sign of writers' block—or any awareness that such a thing exists.[6]

But there's something not quite right. I tell myself it's because of the boardwalk, which tips from side to side as it meanders along the coast— 15km of sloping wooden slats, their supports intermittently sinking as the sandy soil yields to the weight of joggers, bikers, fishermen, young lovers, elderly locals and a variety of purposeful foreign perambulators. If you walk fast enough, it can feel as if you're on a gently rolling ship. Or it could be all the editing, over-taxing my brain and making me dizzy. More likely, I decide, it's the endless barking of the dogs, which forces me to plug my ears at night, pushing the squishy orange cones as deep inside my ears as they will go—and even then I can still hear the high-pitched yapping from the 15 homeless dogs our next-door neighbour has lovingly rescued from the streets and is now housing in his living room. I cannot imagine the chaos of so many boisterous canines colliding in such a small space—not to mention the feeding frenzy, the dog hair, or the furniture, if there's any left.

We should get things checked out, just in case, Lewis tells me. So, after a lunch of grilled sardines, caught fresh this morning, smelly and slithery, from the local fish shop, we head north along the boardwalk to the village of Aguda, 1km away. We pass the salt-water swimming pool and some simple Portuguese dwellings, their open doors yearning for fresh air, and their dark, musty interiors harbouring the vague shapes of plastic-covered tables, cluttered concrete walls and the occasional hunched human wrapped in dark clothing and thick black stockings. Despite the midday May heat that has us sweating in just shorts and T-shirts, the locals consider it cold and wintry until at least late July, and seem to regard our scanty attire as an insult to their superior sensibilities. They don't respond to our greetings or friendly waves (on the rare occasions that they emerge, wearing thick headscarves and shawls) but their traditional timelessness feels reassuring when everything else seems to be shifting like the sand.

Finally, we arrive at the little clinic—a one-storey, white-washed concrete shed with a small waiting area and a single treatment room. The doctor sees us promptly, but she doesn't speak English and I don't speak Portuguese. I try French, Spanish and Italian, but she remains unmoved. She waves over a young man from the waiting area and he interprets for us with unsuppressed delight, as if he's been asked to read the news on TV. I explain the mild hearing loss and the dizziness when walking. The doctor takes a cursory look inside my right ear, humming and hawing to herself, then sits back down behind her desk.

"We do not treat foreigners," says our interpreter, with the appropriate gravitas. "You need special medical card for Portuguese only."

"But can she see anything wrong?" I ask.

"*Não*. Maybe infection? You check with your doctor." He clasps his hands behind his back and rocks on his heels, smiling beneficently as if he's just given us the cure for Alzheimer's.

Feeling medically nonplussed and underwhelmed (a universal condition that can only be self-diagnosed by the most mindful body-owners), we reclaim the sunshine and pause to watch a fisherman pulling nets into an ancient, wooden rowing boat. He is devoted to his task—a ritual that feels like a meditation and makes me want to immerse myself forever in the rhythmic pull of the tides. The sun beats down and the heat fills my body, relaxing muscles, soothing my mind and infusing me with the simple truth that peace can be as easy as breathing in the salty air, succumbing to the waves and allowing myself to be swept away.

"Barbequed fish tonight, with roasted fennel and a glass of your favourite Pinotage?" Lewis asks, putting his arm around me, grounding me and loving me back to reality as only he can do. "I'm cooking."

I smile up at his handsome face, his bright-orange hat contrasting with his dark hair and espresso-bean-coloured eyes, and the moment seems frozen in time and paralysingly precious, as if I must somehow capture its intangible, fleeting blessedness.

"I thought you were going to work on your book," I reply.

"I will," he says, "after dinner."

"I can't wait to see what happens next," I say, knowing that the story is unfolding for him as he writes. I've read all the chapters he's written so far, and I have no idea where it's going.

"A really good gourmet dinner feeds the brain and generates lots of ideas and solutions," he says.

I smile at this as he knows how much I love our chats, and they have generated some fascinating ideas.

"Anyway, I want to savour our time here, and I don't want to know how it ends, just yet," he says.

I love him for trying to distract me so that I don't worry about something that is probably absolutely nothing to worry about.

"We've still got three weeks left," he reminds me—three more weeks of all being deliciously, perfectly well with my world.

2 Trying to find home

I don't know what I'm doing here, back in Ireland—temporarily, I promise myself. I'm missing Vancouver, which has been my home for much of the past two decades, and am intent on returning as soon as I can muster the energy. After touring Europe for almost a year, on a quest for some nice coastline near a small, like-minded community (mission not accomplished), we're regrouping in a townhouse in a quiet *cul de sac*, just a kilometre from my family home. This unexpected geographical detour has thrown me completely off kilter, which may be why I can no longer walk in a straight line.

With its West Coast flavour and progressive, pioneering spirit, Vancouver is much more my kind of place than Ireland. Even though I was raised here, just outside the quaint little village of Dalkey (home to Enya, Chris de Burgh and the late Maeve Binchy, among other notables), it was in Vancouver that I finally grew up. Knee-deep in psychic fertiliser that nourished the dormant seeds of self-expression, I was hungry for an understanding of the mysterious human dynamics that seemed to screw up so many promising lives. But being back in Ireland has tested my hard-won West Coast wisdom, reminding me of the unique power of even the most loving parents to trigger emotional reactions that you thought were a thing of the past.

Now, after all the fruitless travelling, I'm chronologically confused and all over the map. I'm too old to be in this situation, with no home of my own and no investments, and I'm a mishmash of parts that seem to progress in their own sweet time, with no regard for budget, aging or pension. The wise part of me feels ancient and sometimes too intuitive for my own good. Emotionally, I feel quite mature, capable of sane advice and laughing at myself before anyone else does. Financially speaking, however, I'm still in kindergarten, sucking my thumb and hoping for the best; and, when faced with the same old family dynamics that I teach other people how to handle with masterful detachment, I'm still in nappies (aka diapers), prone to tantrums and meltdowns.

But there are plenty of things to keep me distracted. There's a strange buzzing in my head that's been getting louder, over the past few months. Lewis says I think too much, micro-analysing situations when I work with

17

clients on Skype. But that's what they pay me for and I'm good at it. It doesn't feel right, but maybe I've just got to defuse all this electrical over-activity in my brain, drink more water, do more yoga and, above all, stay calm the next time the TV-licence Gestapo send us another letter.

We've already received three letters in the mail, accusing us of secretly harbouring a TV without buying the obligatory licence for it. We haven't owned a TV for over 10 years, but try telling *them* that. That's not normal, they say, and we don't believe you. Come and look, I tell them, but they're convinced I'll just hide it in the garden shed or take it next door till they've gone.

The third letter was the last straw, and I couldn't get to the phone fast enough to enlighten the lovely person who insisted we were TV addicts who were just too cheap to pay the licence fee—despite the fact that I'd written to the licensing office, confirming in no uncertain and only slightly uncharitable terms, that WE DO NOT HAVE any such apparatus in any room, shed, closet, crawl space or attic of our house. Breathing like an escapee from a psychiatric ward, I dial the number and try to compose myself while I wait for someone to answer. I fail utterly and am practically incoherent explaining the reason for my call.

"Are you saying you don't have a TV?" says the female at the other end of the line—someone whose sleuthing skills have clearly been stunted by watching too many soap operas and not enough episodes of CSI.

If she only knew, says The Voice inside my head—the one that talks to me when I worry about things. I've taken to calling it TV and am beginning to think it's even more unhealthy for me to be listening to than the conventional kind, *which you can actually turn off.*

"Yes," I reply, with incredible restraint, *"as I said in my letter."*

"Have you not seen the ads about not buying your licence?" she asks.

"Which ads?" I say, although I know perfectly well what she's referring to, having seen them on my *parents'* TV. They're clever and very funny ...*for people who watch TV.*

"The TV ads," she says.

I want to ask her if she was dropped on her head at birth, but then I wonder if I'm actually speaking to some kind of highly sophisticated answering machine. I assume the former and press on.

"How would I have seen those ads if I don't have a TV?" I reply, gobsmacked by my ability to remain civil, thanks only to my intuitive understanding that I may be dealing with someone who was raised on a diet of fast food, with nowhere near enough essential fatty acids to adequately fuel her brain, and far too many non-essential fatty assets to function properly.

"Listen," I say, generously intervening so she doesn't have to use up precious brain cells trying to figure out the question, "if you send me another threatening letter or if you call me again accusing me of having a TV, I'm going to charge you with harassment. Do you understand?"

"O-kaaay," she says slowly, "but do you really not have a TV?"

For the sake of our mutual sanity, I terminate the call and sit quietly for a moment, contemplating my behaviour. What is going on? Why am I getting so worked up about things? The woman was only doing her job, and this is not the way I usually deal with people.

My head is pounding and I need to lie down. I throw myself on the bed and take some deep breaths. The buzzing in my head starts again, so I hold my breath for as long as I can, several times in a row, and my body finally starts to relax. But then the neighbours' two Boxers start to bark. It's a competitive duet that echoes off the concrete yard where they're strategically penned during the day while the owners are at work, purposely designed to create the maximum acoustic resonance for the house across the street ...which happens to be ours.

I feel as if I want to hit something, which is not my usual style. Why am I so agitated and distraught? I'm feeling so edgy and intolerant that I wonder if I'm cracking up from the strain of being chronically sleep-deprived, zapped and worried about what's going on in my body. I imagine myself turning into a hysterical harridan, slapping the side of my head while screeching maniacally and brandishing a cast-iron frying pan as I chase dogs all over the neighbourhood.

And then I fall asleep.

* * *

A week later, one of the Boxers dies, and I feel a fleeting jolt of guilt. I've been sending dagger-vibes in their direction for the past three months and I'm not surprised to hear that one of them has succumbed. I imagine the vet scratching his head as he examines the body, asking Miriam Dogsbody (I can't remember her surname) if she can account for the multitude of needle punctures all over the riddled corpse. She can't, of course, since she has triple glazing on her windows to ensure that she doesn't hear the constant canine cacophony coming from her beloved boxed-in Boxers, while everyone else has to suffer it, day after dogged day. I love dogs, by the way, and would never harm one, but their incessant barking feels like the last straw for my frazzled nerves.

You can't even get in to her Fort Knox property to talk to her, as the whole place is so heavily walled and neighbour-repellant—which is why I had to write her a letter about her dogs. This did not go down well. When she arrives on our doorstep, as expected, she's spitting venom. I can tell straightaway that Miriam Dogsbody is living up to her pseudonym. She has the brittle air of someone who's having a hard time and desperately needs to vent her anger on someone she feels she can bully ...such as me.

"Hello, Miriam," I say.

"Don't *Miriam* me," she spits. "We're not friends."

I nod in wholehearted agreement.

"How long have you lived here?" she demands. "Do you own this place or are you renting?"

These are personal questions, coming from a non-friend, so I don't feel the need to respond.

"We've lived here for 18 years," she says, her spine straightening, "and I doubt very much you've been here that long." This gives you an indication of how much Miriam interacts with her neighbours. We've only been in this house for six months, in fact. Nonetheless, I grew up in this area and lived nearby till I was 22, so I think I win this particular round.

All that's missing from this conversation is the sandbox and the plastic buckets and spades.

With that image in mind, and given how strange I'm feeling, I realize there's no point in talking further. "Okay!" I say, waving goodbye before closing the door. It wasn't my most powerful comeback ever, but I knew it would not help to fuel the ire of this sad, put-upon woman who seems desperate for some loving human interaction. I feel bad for being so heartless and almost run after her for a proper chat. Maybe I should have given her a nice big anger-deflating hug, but I'm just so tired and I can't seem to summon the energy to initiate a more compassionate conversation. This disturbs me, as I can sense that she's troubled and, like everyone else, in need of some validation. I would normally have been more understanding. After all, I'm a therapist, for heaven's sake, and I know better than to behave this way, so now I feel sorry for us both.

I decide to do some housework, but only because it's a productive way of alleviating my angst. I start with the bathroom, scrubbing the sinks like the dutiful housewife that I'm not (but it's good practice for the leading role I'm hoping to play in a movie some day). I'm finding lots of my blond hairs, which is annoying, but manageably so. Lewis's hairs, on the other hand, are *everywhere*—short, dark ones that have colonized every inch of the house, infiltrated all my clothes, and have no doubt left a thick trail all over Europe. I'm thinking they could form the basis for an alternative *El Camino*—a soft, keratinaceous carpet revered by barefooted pilgrims everywhere. I imagine the hairs going stratospheric, floating around the cosmos and puzzling astronomers who cannot figure out where all these tiny black filaments have come from.

But then I get another bout of electrical buzzing in my head, which, regrettably, puts an end to housework for the day. It's getting worse (the buzzing and, consequently, the housework), fragmenting my sleep and distracting me from the rest of my life (i.e., the remainder of my life, as opposed to the best rest of my life, although *that's* true, too). I think it's also affecting my brain, since I seem to have developed a compulsion for speaking in really long sentences, with lots of clauses, em dashes and parentheses. A certain amount of insomnia is okay. I can amuse myself for hours as I lie awake at night—making up new words, writing my Oscar acceptance speech for best documentary, and inventing 10 creative uses for knee socks—but it would be better for my health (not to mention my sanity and longevity) if I could get more sleep. (*See what I mean?*) Plus, the buzzing is starting to worry me.

I think I know what's causing it and I need to talk to Lewis. It feels like an electrical jolt from a baby Taser, and it started after we got the WiMAX antenna installed on our roof—right above our bedroom. How could I ever have agreed to such a thing? Having a high-powered radiation signal beaming into our home, day and night, makes no sense. *What was I thinking?*

I find Lewis in the conservatory, painting. It's probably not the best time to discuss this, but it suddenly feels urgent.

"I don't think we should have that antenna on the roof," I say. "I think it's affecting me."

"I need the WiFi for my work," Lewis says, stepping back to squint at his canvas. (We realize later that this is not true, of course. We don't need WiFi— aka wireless radiation; we just need an Internet connection, safely hard-wired from a modem to our laptops.)

He's doing an extraordinary painting that I already love—a reclining nude in a vibrant mix of marbled orange, canary-yellow and copper skin tones, rendered with his usual talented translation of form and feeling.[7]

"But we don't have to use that system," I say. "We can get something else."

"We decided that this was the best deal, with the fastest speed. Remember?"

I do, but how can I be held accountable for that when I was clearly out of my mind, at the time? I still am, apparently, if my recent behaviour is anything to go by.

"I still think we should switch," I say, feeling uneasy.

"We paid a lot for the antenna and the installation," Lewis reminds me. "Let's wait a bit and see if you keep having problems. Okay?" He's focusing on his painting and I can see that the topic is closed—for him, at least.

I walk away, feeling conflicted. I don't want the stress of forcing the issue and then dealing with the logistics of getting the antenna removed, paying the penalty fee and finding another service-provider, but I feel twinges of fear and defeat, as if there's an inevitability about the whole thing that is beyond my power to change. I promise myself that I'll bring it up again, a week from now.

3 Inklings of decline

"She was unique," Lewis is saying to the crowd gathered around him. "She was nutty, inventive and endlessly, annoyingly creative, with an imagination and irreverent humour that kept me in a constant state of creative angst and helpless laughter.

"She was the quirkiest person I've ever met. Every day, she came up with a new word or joke, a unique and powerful way of looking at things and profound insights that made sense of all the craziness in our world. There are so many things about her that I will remember—so many aspects of life that she nailed with her wisdom and humour that I don't know how I can face any more Olga-less days without that multi-dimensional madness.

"I have so many images of her in my head. She always cut her oranges in half and gnawed at the flesh like a savage, juice running down her chin. If I brought home lamb burgers, she'd make Lamburghinis, warning me not to expect *fast* food. She called me chairman of the ironing board when I ironed my shirts at the weekend, because I'm also the chairman for a non-profit organization.

"She had fears and insecurities of her own, even though she helped so many others overcome theirs, and whenever she managed to do a presentation or handle some important issue in a powerful way, she'd spontaneously shout *I did it!* every few hours, wherever she happened to be, for at least a week.

"She had a favourite large kitchen spoon that she used for everything, except one particularly challenging task that required a bit more dexterity and a smaller utensil. It involved detaching what she called the *umbilicals* when she cracked eggs for omelettes. She had a violent aversion to these bits of the egg and would gag and dry-retch histrionically every time she spooned them into the sink. The eggs had to be cooked properly, too, as she wouldn't eat them if they were what she called *frilly*. No moving parts, she said.

"Although she had an innate elegance, no matter what she wore, she was messy in many ways, with terrible handwriting and a desk diary that was filled with indecipherable hieroglyphics. Yet she had a mind like a steel trap and an ability to pick up on details that no normal person would ever notice or care about. She could read people and she often made allowances for them, even if they treated her badly, as she could understand the source of their pain

22

or anger. She had more integrity than this world deserves and was forever questioning her own actions, reactions and motives for doing things.

"She was humble about her abilities, yet wildly enthusiastic about mine, dedicated to helping me be more me. She saved my life, showing me—"

Darn! He was just getting to a good bit. I sit up in bed, disappointed to find out that this poignant eulogy is a dream and that the world did not, in fact, get to hear my lovely husband tell them how amazing I am …*was*. I feel devastated that I'm not dead and the focus of all that devotion, but then I realize the idiocy of this thought and remind myself that the source of that devotion is currently downstairs in the kitchen, painstakingly and lovingly removing the *umbilicals* from my eggs.

As I'm getting dressed and putting on my socks (since I can't wear my favourite flip-flops on this sodding soggy island), I notice that my hands are shaking. I pause to reflect, and I realize that I've been in a constant state of agitation since… I can't remember when. These days, I can't seem to relax. It's as if my body has been on speed (or is perpetually high on chocolate) and is going through withdrawal. Inside, I feel shaky, nervous, jittery and filled with a free-floating anxiety that has no reason to be there. *What is happening to me?* The eulogy that Lewis just gave me (or I imagined him giving me) reminds me of my more stable, healthy self, and I sense that my personality has changed in subtle, incremental ways that I hadn't noticed until now. *I must remember all those things that he (through me) just said about me*, I decide. A pre-mortem eulogy provides a precious reminder of all that we aspire to be, before it's too late to recapture ourselves. I think everyone should have one.

I hurry downstairs, eager to thank Lewis for his wonderful words, but I catch myself on the last step. I know he already thinks I'm nuts (he just said so, didn't he?), but thanking him for an imaginary eulogy might be pushing things a bit, so I restrain myself. I want to write one for him, though, now that I know how nice it is to be showered with post-humous praise while you're still alive to hear it. The only thing worse than not being around to hear the tribute paid to you by the person you love is for him (or her) to not be around to hear theirs.

Just a few hours later, I get some news that brings death much closer to home. The 21-year-old son of one of my best friends has died suddenly and tragically, at their home, just a few kilometres away. This hits me with almost physical force, making me so wobbly I can hardly walk.

As I absorb this shocking news, I'm aware of being so depleted that it's hard for me to handle any additional trauma. It will be another few years before I realize that ongoing exposure to microwave radiation (which accumulates in the body, over time) has worn me down and left me with little resilience for everyday living, not to mention tragedies such as this.

4 Feeling the fields and losing our connection

For as long as I can remember, shopping malls have made me feel ill. It's not the shopping that affects me, although things *can* get a bit intense when you're looking for natural cotton clothing and you're surrounded by electrifying polyester, clingy rayon and frilly nylon stuff. Within 10 minutes of entering a shopping mall, or any large shop (especially one selling electronics), I feel dizzy, nauseous and light-headed. I rapidly dehydrate, with waves of heat going up and down my body. I can no longer think straight, walk straight or do any more shopping. I head home as fast as I can, and it takes me at least two days to recver from the effects. Please bear this in mind if you ever see me out and about, looking a bit scruffy and less than well-dressed. It's hard to do any good-quality shopping in under 10 minutes.

It was a long time before I realized that I was reacting to the high levels of electromagnetic fields (EMFs) in shops and high-rise buildings. As with so many of the symptoms caused by electromagnetic radiation, I attributed my reaction to other things. I was sure I had some as-yet-undiagnosed condition. (I did, but not the kind I suspected.) I was convinced I had some kind of immune disorder, a nervous-system disorder, or maybe even some kind of slow-growing cancer that would only reveal itself when it was too late to do anything about it. I wasn't hoping for that. I just wanted an explanation for the way I was feeling.

Finding none, I blamed everything else I could think of: my diet (even though I have arguably one of the world's best-fed and most expensively nourished bodies); my lifestyle, which was pretty good, as I walked or biked everywhere, did yoga and was as active as I could be; my work, which I loved and which nourished and inspired me in many ways; my emotional state, which was fairly balanced, with a healthy quotient of craziness and only the occasional bout of mundane normalcy, countered by lots of laughter, positive thinking and affirmative action; and my relationships, which included an exceptional hubby, fabulous siblings, some wonderful friends, and supportive, loving parents.

What the heck...? Nothing made sense. I poured thousands of dollars into various therapies that might make me better, and spent years researching supplements and information that might fix this persistent problem. Going to the doctor for various tests only made me feel worse, and it wasn't just their lack of awareness or their obsession with pharmaceutical drugs. (*Say NO! to drugs*, I tell them, but they can't seem to break free.) It was also the overhead fluorescent lights (ubiquitous in all medical facilities, despite the fact that they emit radiation), which I finally realized were giving me headaches and making me feel unwell.

I was becoming more and more fatigued and aging alarmingly fast. *Ah. Of course*, proclaimed those same wise physicians. *It's your hormones!* As the years progressed, doctors began trotting out the inevitable universal explanation for anything that ailed a woman over 40: *it's that time of life*, they'd say, patting my hand pityingly. I was getting older, so I had to *expect* this kind of thing as my hormones diminished. But I'd been feeling this way for a very long time (although getting progressively worse) so, if they were right, I must have hit menopause over a decade ago, without realizing it. It was a nice story, but I wasn't buying it. I was desperate for answers, but not *that* desperate. I could not override my own reasoning, research and intuitive sense that this was not right.

I think of this now and I realize that this is what it's like for so many people all over the world—all desperately trying to find the reason for their illness and never suspecting that it's coming right at them, permeating their cells, penetrating their bones and irradiating every aspect of their existence. Ironically, many of them use their cell phones to research their health issues and to comfort themselves by texting friends and checking for e-mails or messages on Facebook.

Our deep need for human connection blinds us to many things, including our innate worthiness and lovability, which often results in us not getting the closeness we seek. We can only be emotionally complete and self-sufficient if we are emotionally, physically and spiritually nourished, with meaningful relationships and a heartfelt commitment to be true to ourselves. Being emotionally whole means enhancing our self-worth to the point where we feel deeply deserving of love, support and validation, which enables us to powerfully express and embrace our authentic selves, with no need for approval or permission from others.

I think of the tragic death of my friend's young son, who had felt emotionally isolated and tried to resolve his emotional issues by self-medicating with herbs he purchased online. That loss of human connection costs us dearly, and it shows up in many ways, with a disturbing increase in the incidence of young children attempting or contemplating suicide. What does this say about us, as parents, teachers, siblings and friends, when children as young as 10 are calling suicide help lines?[8]

As my tolerance for EMFs decreases and I become increasingly isolated from others, I get plenty of time to ponder this issue. Plus, it's central to my work, which explores human dynamics—why we do the things we do and what drives us to be the people we are. Since so much of what drives us is buried in our subconscious, dating back to our early, formative years, most of us remain unaware of the fears and beliefs that shape our reality. We don't realize the power of those beliefs or how they determine the risks we take, our reactions to things, the insecurities and expectations we have, the things we accept without question, the degree to which we defer to others, the compromises we make for the sake of acceptance, and so many other things that we assume are just an integral part of who we are or the way life is.

5 Pressure increasing

The hard metal chairs are not conducive to lingering, lounging or even sitting upon—not that we feel inclined to do any of these things in this disturbingly soulless place. It's a miracle that we found the right room—or, more accurately, the third cubicle in the right-hand corner of the fifth room on the left, off the second corridor on your right at the top of the middle stairwell on the fourth floor. A seemingly endless warren of echoey rooms with high ceilings, sickly-blue walls, and Formica-topped desks behind milky-grey room-dividers, it feels like a prison that was re-purposed when all the inmates died of sensory deprivation. Or maybe they just got lost and killed themselves in despair, realizing that they would never again see another friendly prison guard, enjoy the satisfyingly smooth texture of the morning gruel, or hear the reassuring cries of their lunatic comrades as they thrashed around on their cozy steel bunks at night—

"It's a small benign tumour—an acoustic neuroma," says Mr Pierce, pointing at the MRI scan of my skull, and bringing me back to the present, where I really don't want to be. "It's not cancerous, though, so no need to worry."

I lean forward, looking at the computer monitor in front of us. The consultant—*not even a doctor*, I tell myself, as if that might somehow invalidate his diagnosis—is confirming what I already suspected. After grudgingly taking antibiotics for the non-existent *infection* and getting a CT scan that (they failed to tell me) emitted over 1,000 times more radiation than a standard x-ray yet failed to reveal anything at all, I'm finally coming face to face with the real culprit—clearly, undeniably, horribly evident on the screen just two feet away.

Excellent, I think: a tumour that's growing on a cranial nerve, inside my ear, snuggling up to my brain, making me dizzy, making me walk funny and making me deaf. But it's not cancerous, so why *would* I worry? Plus, it's only 2cm big and there's plenty of space in my head for something that small.

"Ms Sheean…"

He interrupts my thoughts …gain. Does he not understand that I need to digest this and that it takes time for me to adjust to my entire world having tilted on its axis, and to decide whether I want to actually *accept* what he's telling me? And how dare he tell me I've got a tumour without even giving me a proper consulting room with four walls and a closable door.

"Do you understand what I'm saying?"

He thinks I'm in shock. I'm not feeling well, but it's the effect of this place. The walls exude a kind of historical halitosis—generations of stinky emanations that force you to shallow-breathe. The air is so clogged that you have to practically beat it with your fists to make room for your next sentence.

"Yes," I say, but there's so much resistance that the word bounces back and hits me in the face. I look pointedly at Lewis. *See?* I take a deep breath and give it more oomph. "YES!" This time, it manages to get through and Mr Perry flinches from the impact.

He turns his attention to my file, checking to see if there's any family history of psychosis or early dementia, and I'm struck by the inherent *wrongness* of it all. I'm surrounded by the inertia of inevitability—patients blindly accepting what they're told, almost like robots, with no sense of being in charge of their own lives. With no airtime for the body's own wisdom, there's no joyful anticipation of true health and vitality—no one whistling jauntily down the corridor, thrilled to have regained their health, due to the miracles of modern medicine. It's as if everyone's being inoculated with a dose of bad news, with a complimentary side order of pessimism, and a full menu of medical misdirection offering a smorgasbord of drugs and symptom control.

There's a strange woman staring straight at me through the gap between the room dividers. I glare at her and she slowly turns away, at the desultory speed of 200mg of lithium a day, like a massive ocean liner trying to change course in a sea of thick mud, or a—

Mr Pierce, Mr Plant, or whatever this non-doctor is called, is now telling me what might or might not happen, but that I shouldn't worry, either way.

"There are three possible approaches," he is saying, enunciating slowly, as if talking to a witless child. "We can do surgery, although there's no need for that yet; we can try some drugs that might help with the symptoms; or we can adopt the wait-and-see approach."

We? I don't think it's going to help me if he takes the drugs, too. And what kind of approach is 'waiting and seeing'? How can doing nothing be an approach? That woman is staring at me again and I want to— But Mr Petty intervenes, unwittingly saving her from a searing, lethal look, which could have left her emotionally scarred for the rest of her life and in need of ongoing therapy to deal with the trauma.

"Ms Sheean," he says, "there's no cause for immediate concern."

I give him a piercing look, which seems fair enough to me, if his name is Pierce, although I'm less sure about this, now that I think about it. He should be wearing a nametag so I don't have to waste precious brain power remembering such things when I'm grappling with mind-numbing news.

"Is there cause for slightly *delayed* concern?"

He continues as if I haven't just asked him a perfectly valid question.

"These things tend to grow very slowly, and it could be years before it becomes a real problem."

I study this man and wonder what planet he's from, and what he did to deserve being relegated to the airless nether-regions of this former prison for the mentally deranged. Or maybe he's one of the former inmates and they kept him on because he knew his way around.

I force myself to focus on the more immediate matter of the rest of my life. "It's *already* a real problem," I tell him, since he seems to be exceptionally dim—possibly because he never had any medical training, or maybe because he *did*. "How do you know that mine grew slowly?" I challenge him. "It might have started growing last year and look at the size of it now! It's already 2cm and could be growing like crazy, even as we speak, and you wouldn't know."

Lewis puts a calming hand on my knee and I glare at him as lovingly as can be expected, given the circumstances. I turn to glare less lovingly at that woman, ready to give her the full whack of my most potent, searing scowl, but she's gone—back to her life of lovely lithium-laced tumour-free tomorrows.

"Ms Sheean," Mr Pratt is saying, "it's very unlikely that yours grew that fast. These neuromas normally take years to develop and it's not always necessary to do anything about them, as long as they don't interfere with normal life."

I want to ask this man if walking like a drunkard, feeling dizzy and progressively losing your hearing are part of his normal life, but he's Irish, so they might be—if he drinks a lot, gets hung-over and has the kind of nutritional deficiencies that cause age-related hearing loss. I decide it would be more productive to enlighten him about the real impact of this tumour, from the perspective of someone who actually has one, versus someone who can only theorize about them from a place of superior smugness, safe in the knowledge that their brain is not being shoved aside by a rapidly growing 'neuromatic' monster.

But Lewis squeezes my knee and I realize the insanity of trying to reason with a former inmate of this former prison for the criminally insane. I thank Mr Pringle for his time, gather up my coat and the MRI printout, and walk as steadily as I can, without meandering too much, towards the maze that, if correctly navigated, will take us to the exit of Dublin's illustrious St James Hospital.

Lewis guides me with his usual unerring sense of direction, finally delivering us back into the open air, where we pause to recalibrate and adjust to the radical shift in our universe. It feels as if we've been through a time warp.

"That went well, don't you think?" He almost makes me smile. I hug him fiercely, soaking up his solid, loving presence—my safest place on the planet—and I exhale for the first time since entering the Tardis of St James five years ago this morning. Then I start to laugh and I can't stop. I laugh until tears stream down my face and Lewis is looking at me as if I've lost my mind—which I'm perfectly entitled to do, thank you very much, since the whole world has apparently gone mad. But it's not the tumour that's making me hysterical. I think of our 1990 Fiat Punto parked nearby and I'm wondering how much the parking fine will be after being gone for five years.

I laugh all the way back to the car, telling myself that it's better than crying.

The crying will come later, says TV—that mutinous voice inside my head, the squatter in my skull, which has really been getting on my cranial nerves. *Plenty of time for that.* I stop short and answer it back, determined to nip this one in the bud: "Listen, you free-loading leech…" but Lewis is eyeing me with concern, probably wondering if I've been affected by the madness lingering within the walls of St James. And maybe I have been. I'm aware that my crazy sense of humour is the only thing keeping me sane, even though it probably makes me sound completely nuts.

I smile reassuringly at Lewis as he unlocks the car, then quickly finish up with The Voice: *Any more of that toxic negative thinking and I'll flood you with every pharmaceutical drug in existence. I die, you die. So just zip it, okay?*

TV is suitably subdued and remains quiet for the rest of the journey home.

6 There goes the neighbourhood

We're back in Vancouver after our valiant attempt to live the good life in Ireland. I love my Irish friends (and family, too, of course), but even love isn't enough to make up for the climate. Fix the wretched weather over there and we'll come back for an annual visit (although given how I felt after the last long-haul flight, I'm not sure I can keep that promise). In the absence of reliable stretches of restorative sunshine, I'm too cranky to endure chronic corrosion from all that wet stuff, and drowning my sorrows in alcohol just doesn't work for me. I do admire the perpetual Irish optimism, though. Hoping for sunshine, despite decades of dismal rainy summers, shows a strength of character that I seem to lack. Or maybe it's just a necessary kind of self-delusion that makes living there possible.

Not that Vancouver doesn't get its fair share of rain, but at least it seems to be mostly restricted to a few months of the year, often coming in Monsoon-like downpours that go on for days. But I'll take the short-and-sweet deluge over ongoing drizzle any day. The summers are long and hot, giving you plenty of time to completely dry out and work up some healthy-looking freckles.

I'm glad to be back. It's my third time living here—alternating with two stints in Switzerland and our recent European odyssey—and I've officially decided that this is my favourite place to live.

Living where we do, in my favourite part of the city, we have easy access to everything. With its tree-lined streets, abundant greenery spilling over the footpaths, lovingly tended gardens with rockeries and even benches for passersby to sit on, a unique assortment of colourful wooden houses, several beaches within walking distance, mountains in the background, and all the amenities and healthfoods you need just a few blocks away, funky Kitsilano is *the* place to be. Having sold our car before returning to Europe, we now bike everywhere, which is easy to do on the many designated bike paths.

The downside of all this aesthetically pleasing, effortless, eco-friendly living is that lots of other people want to live here, too. The city is booming, with a growing number of wealthy immigrants inflating the cost of housing and changing the whole cultural vibe. It's a far cry from the laid-back bohemian place I fell in love with when I first moved here in 1992.

There are lots of young people, which gives the city a dynamic feel, with lots of learning going on and lots of boisterous young bodies playing volleyball on the beach. There's activity everywhere—people out on bikes, cruising in their convertibles, jogging along the sea wall, huddled conspiratorially in crowded cafés, dashing off to business meetings, talking importantly on their phones as they beetle along in their snappy suits and $300 Fluevog shoes, out walking with hip baby-strollers (the babies being almost an accessory), dragging their toy Poodle on a leash—everyone cheerful and vivaciously buoyant. Out shopping, you're bound to see something gossip-worthy—a man in a clown suit riding a unicycle down 4th Avenue, a huge parrot chained to the steering wheel of an old Jag convertible, and a seemingly destitute homeless person collecting bottles for the recycling refund …who then gets into her spanking-new SUV and drives off.

I love it. But, even as I'm living it, it begins to slowly recede as I find myself less and less able to engage. All the cafés are noisy and now offer free WiFi. Going downtown to do some shopping is no longer fun or even mildly tolerable. Even being on the beach is no longer the peaceful retreat that it once was, due to all the cell phones that everyone *must* carry or something awful might happen (such as missing an important call from their spouse asking if he should buy white bread or brown). Meanwhile, my friends are flying high—attending seminars, giving seminars, joining Meet-ups, jet-setting off to Mexico, skiing in Whistler, going to see movies, meeting up for dinner in some chic downtown tapas bar, and generally living life to the max …and reporting it all on Facebook.

Within six months of our return, I'm floundering. The tumour is growing and I'm feeling constant cranial pressure and tension. The buzzing continues and the dehydration is adding even more years to my face. I've had to ease back on my work and I'm spending a lot of time alone, doing yoga, riding my bike to the beach, picking up books from the library... I'm doing all I can to reverse the growth but my body seems unable to oblige. With a creeping sense of dread, I'm beginning to doubt my ability to heal myself.

7 What you need to know about electromagnetic radiation and electro-sensitivity

As parents, we strive to keep our children safe, doing our best to be emotionally available, to protect them from bullying, abuse and second-hand smoke, and to feed them nutritious food. Yet here we are, causing untold harm to our youngest and most vulnerable, walking around with cell phones, while carrying our babies in a body sling. We're exposing our youths and teenagers to harmful microwave radiation—not just at home but in schools, libraries and almost every other public place. And we're wired for sound (and visuals and games) in every square foot of our homes and offices.

Looking back at past generations, we may find it hard to believe that doctors used to promote cigarettes as being good for our health, and that tapeworms were sold as a great way to lose weight. Sadly, it's only in retrospect that we can see our own 'blind spots'. What will the next generation think of us, when it becomes widely recognized that our high-tech radiation-emitting gadgets are creating all kinds of health problems and fatal illnesses—not to mention killing off the birds and bees so essential to our food supply?

What is electromagnetic hypersensitivity (EHS)?

Electromagnetic hypersensitivity (also referred to as electro-sensitivity) is an environmentally induced condition resulting from the electromagnetic fields (EMFs) and radio-frequency (RF) waves that permeate our living and working environments. Both are forms of non-ionizing radiation that affect all forms of life, even at extremely low levels. This radiation causes a biologically verifiable reaction that occurs at a cellular level, affecting the blood and causing a multitude of symptoms and conditions[9] that are often attributed to other causes or remain undiagnosed.

How much we are affected by EMFs depends on our resilience, degree and duration of exposure, stress levels, lifestyle, genetics and other factors. Many individuals seem unaffected (or are unaware of being affected) and dismiss electro-sensitivity as invalid. Yet, according to Dr Erica Mallery-Blythe, a former accident-and-emergency doctor now specializing in EHS, many of us may be electro-hypersensitive and not realize it. "Everybody has the potential to become electro-hypersensitive," she says, "[since] every cell in our body, in our brain or nervous system is dependent on electrical signals."[10]

First described in 1932, electro-sensitivity (known then as radiowave or microwave sickness) tends to worsen with continued exposure, creating a vicious circle: ongoing exposure reduces one's tolerance, which leads to an increase in symptoms, when then further reduces one's tolerance.

Key physical effects of man-made electromagnetic radiation[11]

1. Nervous system disruption, which sends the body into a perpetual fight-or-flight response and prevents it from resting, repairing, healing or regenerating normally.

2. Reduced production of melatonin—the body's sleep hormone, required for healthy sleep cycles. Melatonin is also anti-carcinogenic and the body's only natural antioxidant. When it is depleted, it causes oxidative stress and accelerated aging due to harmful free radicals.

3. Impaired immune system, in the form of decreased natural killer cells and other white-blood-cell damage.

4. Reproductive problems, such as sterility, infertility issues and hormonal disruption.

5. Breakdown of the blood–brain barrier, causing the death of neurons and the leakage of toxins into the brain, which can lead to early dementia, Alzheimer's disease, Attention Deficit Hyperactivity Disorder (ADHD) and autism.

6. Increased cerebral glucose metabolism, also linked to Alzheimer's (known as 'diabetes of the brain').

7. DNA damage, the effects of which include an increased risk of cancer and a loss of fertility.[12]

8. Oxidative stress and chronic inflammation, which affect all the body's organs, causing numerous degenerative and other conditions such as cancer, diabetes, osteoporosis, heart disease, rapid aging and arthritis.

9. Inhibition of repair mechanisms, preventing the body from recovering or healing normally.

10. Disruption of voltage-gated calcium channels, which results in the leaching of calcium and the opening of the various tight junction barriers in our bodies that normally protect us from allergens and toxins in the environment, preventing toxic materials in the bloodstream from entering sensitive parts of the body such as the brain.[13]

11. Production of heat-shock proteins, in response to a wide variety of stressors, including weak electromagnetic fields; these proteins act as "chaperones to protect important enzymes", says Dr Andrew Goldsworthy, but continued exposure to EMFs can deplete the body's protective mechanisms.

12. Interference with the body's cellular communication.

13. Disruption of circadian rhythms—the body's natural cycles of sleep and wakefulness.

According to French oncologist Dr Dominique Belpomme, who specializes in treating those with EHS,[14] "The first phase is induced by exposure to a specific EMF frequency—either an acute or chronic exposure, such as talking on a cell phone 20 minutes every day. The first signs of hypersensitivity [due to cell phone use] are pain and a heat sensation in the ear. In the second phase, the disease sets in. That's when you become intolerant at all frequencies."

The symptoms of EHS include but are not limited to the following:

- Insomnia/sleep disturbances
- Headaches, sharp pains, tingling, numbness
- Pressure in head/throat/chest/ears, tinnitus
- Dizziness, balance issues
- Electrical buzzing or 'zapping' in head
- Visual/hearing disturbances, eye irritation
- Short-term memory loss, mental block, concentration problems
- Skin rashes, eczema
- Cancer

- Brain fog and impaired cognitive function
- Neurological, digestive, metabolic and immune disorders
- Chronic dehydration, insatiable thirst
- Altered heart rate, palpitations, heart issues, blood pressure anomalies
- Tremors, tics, seizures
- Extreme fatigue
- Joint dysfunction, musculoskeletal pains
- Increased chemical sensitivity and/or allergies
- induced fight-or-flight response, post-traumatic stress disorder
- Sensory overload, inability to rest/relax/heal

While this might seem like an improbably long list, it makes sense that all body functions/systems can potentially be affected, given how the radiation affects the body at the cellular level.

If you're experiencing any of these symptoms, it may *not* be because of exposure to microwave or other forms of electromagnetic radiation. However, the likelihood of your symptoms being caused or exacerbated by EMR is increasing every day, even though most of the effects go misdiagnosed, undiagnosed and/or are 'treated' with drugs. According to Dr Mallery-Blythe, some features of EHS require emergency management, such as seizures, cardiac chest pain and malignant arrhythmias, among others. There are also some hallmark signs of EHS, she says, such as body hotspots with increased sensitivity (such as the right ear, from using a cell phone, or the right hand, from using a computer mouse); chemical sensitivity; and a temporary relief from symptoms by bathing/showering, which has a grounding effect on the body.

When we understand that the body is a highly sensitive electromagnetic system, we realize why exposing it to artificial, man-made electromagnetic fields is not a good idea.

While many are not aware of being affected by this ambient manmade radiation, those who *are* aware are said to be having a biologically correct reaction. Our electromagnetic bodies are designed to resonate with the Earth's natural electromagnetic frequency, also known as the Schumann resonance— the natural heartbeat of the Earth. This frequency used to be 7.83 hertz, although that appears to be changing.[15] The Earth's natural frequencies have a healing, grounding effect, and exposure to unnatural EMFs is guaranteed to disrupt the natural order of things.

Electromagnetic radiation is coming at us from every angle—from cell phones, cordless phones, WiFi networks, smart meters, laptops, wireless keyboards/printers, kitchen appliances, electronic equipment, heating systems and fluorescent lights. (See Appendix 1 for a summary of the common sources of man-made electromagnetic radiation in our environment.) Microwave radiation from wireless devices is now so pervasive in our urban and even rural environments that we can no longer avoid being exposed to it.

Not only that, but often the wiring in a house or building can contain what is known as dirty electricity—radio-frequency and electromagnetic interference that produces magnetic fields that emanate from the walls into our living space. Dirty electricity comes from lots of different sources—our power lines, dimmer switches and electrical appliances (especially those with a transformer).[16]

All modern electronic devices—computers, TVs, stereo equipment, CFL bulbs and low-voltage lights—use transformers to convert our relatively clean 60Hz AC electricity to the low-voltage power they use.

To save energy, these transformers 'chop up' the alternating current supply, using it in short bursts as opposed to a smooth continuous flow. This constant stopping and starting of the electrical current causes a combination of what engineers call *electrical feedback*—known in technical terms as *electrical transients* and *harmonics*. This electrical pollution rides along on a building's electrical system with the ability to contaminate an entire home and even buildings and homes nearby.

Dirty electricity has the potential to cause numerous conditions, such as chronic fatigue syndrome, allergies, depression, Alzheimer's disease, Parkinson's disease, Lou Gehrig's disease, attention deficit disorder, cancer, infertility, miscarriage and birth defects.

I learned quite a bit from Jim Waugh's fascinating book on EMR (*Living Safely with Electromagnetic Radiation*[17]), which is an eye-opener for those seeking an explanation for their health-related conundrums. Over the years, Jim has done countless EMF assessments and he shares the stories of individuals whose debilitating conditions disappeared when the source of electromagnetic radiation was detected and removed. Pets, too, can be seriously affected, with dogs, cats, horses and other animals succumbing to lameness, tumours, diarrhoea, skin diseases and paralysis—often because of a cordless phone in their owner's home.

Already painfully aware of the harm that EMFs can do, I need no further convincing of the importance of further 'cleaning up my act'. For most people, though, it's an 'inconvenient truth' and they won't see the need to 'fix' something that they don't consider to be a problem. We all love our mobility-enhancing wireless devices, and very few will willingly give them up.

I decide to get Jim to do an EMF assessment of our home, which is the two lower floors of an older wooden house, owned by the woman living in the two floors above us. The assessment is done in late 2012, shortly before the electricity smart meter got turned on. At the time, the meter is not emitting microwave radiation, and we only realize much later that it was activated sometime in early 2013. At around the same time, the owner switches to another Internet service-provider and, unbeknownst to us at the time, boosts her WiFi system.

Jim takes readings of the radio-frequency/microwave radiation levels throughout our home, pointing out the hot spots and the areas we need to address. In our laundry room, which is beside our bedroom and right below our kitchen, he finds high levels of magnetic fields coming from some ungrounded wiring. The wiring comes from the landlady's apartment above us and, as Jim explains, it emits the kind of magnetic fields known to cause leukemia and many other serious conditions.

Lewis and I exchange looks when we hear this, knowing how our landlady is likely to react if we share this information with her. She's not open to this kind of thing. If it can't be seen, smelt or touched, it's dismissed as nonsense. She thinks we're *fussy* and *difficult*—despite the fact that we've helped her with various things around the house and garden.

She's not interested in what I call the ABCs of life—acceptance (the healthy self-accepting kind, not the *accepting-my-fate* or *being-a-doormat* kind), boundaries (the kind that demonstrate our healthy self-worth and prevent others from mistreating us), and compassion (which I must cultivate for myself and for anyone I fail to understand). But I don't mean to sound superior or to diminish her, since I have yet to fully master these three qualities myself. I couldn't, anyway. I've learned that we can never diminish another person and, if we try to, we just end up diminishing ourselves. How we treat others says more about us than it does about them.

However, she does own this $4m house in which we're living, so I don't feel *too* sorry for her, and she seems to enjoy loud rock music on the weekends, till very late at night—as we know from the thumping reverberations throughout our home, which has zero sound insulation. We've talked to her about this, as it prevented me from sleeping (which is already challenging enough), and this is apparently one of the many things that make us *fussy* and *difficult*.

Given our track record with the landlady, I don't relish the idea of telling her about the harmful electrical currents. My ex-husband's niece died of leukemia at the age of 14—and her home was very close to electricity pylons (aka *power towers*). I don't doubt the connection. Research has revealed a correlation between leukemia and proximity to electricity pylons.[18] Now, years later, having done so much more research, I don't doubt the science behind it, either.

We finally tell our landlady about what Jim found, but she isn't buying it. There will be no electrician coming to fix the wiring and eliminate the harmful EMFs—and we can't even pay one to do the work for us. They all refuse to do any electrical work without the owner's permission.

Ignorance is bliss, they say, but I don't think so. Ignorance is at the root of almost everything that ails us. It is why we get sick, why we get stuck, why we get divorced, why we get cancer, why we eat the wrong stuff, why we abuse our bodies, why we misunderstand each other, why we have conflicts and wars, and why we all seem to need painful wake-up calls in order to figure out what's really going on. So, you can just EMF off with your frigging blissful ignorance. (I don't mean you, lovely reader. I'm talking about certain property-owners who appear to know as much about science as they do about good music—but I'm probably just being ignorant. In fact, I'm as ignorant about her as she is about me and, sadly, she has no interest in sitting down with us for a chat, as we've suggested.)

Ignorance is also why I fail to realize, at the time, that our decision to compromise and not to force the issue ends up costing me a lot more than I could have imagined. While I focused on the microwave radiation coming from wireless devices, I had no idea that magnetic fields could cause just as much damage.

How to minimize the negative impact of EMFs in your home

These are some of the tips Jim gave us:

- **Never leave an unused appliance plugged in**, as the cord/cable and socket will emit a strong electrical field. Don't stand near them, either, when in use.

- **Stand back from the electric elements on your stove**, when turned on. They too emit a strong electrical field.

- **Change all your so-called energy-saving CFLs back to incandescent bulbs**—if you can, as they can be hard to find, given that CFL bulbs are heavily promoted as the more eco-friendly option. CFLs emit harmful radiation (causing skin burns if placed too close to the body), and they contain toxic mercury. According to Walt McGinnis, a licensed journeyman electrician with extensive experience in electromagnetic radiation, CFLs actually increase a consumer's carbon footprint because they are energy hogs to produce, operate and dispose of (See http://bit.ly/2dHbnef).

- **Never sleep with an electrical cable or plug behind or near your head**—such as the cord from a bedside lamp going behind your bed to reach a socket. The electrical field can disrupt sleep and other body functions. Check the other side of your bedroom wall for any appliances plugged in there, for the same reason.

- **Use a separate wired keyboard with your laptop**, if possible. Using the built-in keyboard exposes you to a strong electrical field.

- **Switch from a cordless phone to a corded one.** This may not be easy or convenient to do, but numerous health problems have been associated with the use of cordless phones—among pets as well as humans. Cordless phones use the same kind of pulsed microwave radiation as cell phones and are known to be more dangerous because they operate 24 hours a day, even when the handset is not in use. Unlike cell phones, they never power down and the base is like a tiny cell tower, emitting high levels of radiation that extends in all directions for 100 feet or more.

- **Hard-wire your modem/router to your computer** and turn off the WiFi function—or, at the very least, turn off WiFi at night and when not in use.

- **Keep your cell phone switched off when not in use.** Never wear it on your person and never charge it or keep it in your bedroom at night. During the day, avoid putting it in a breast/hip pocket. Keep cell phones away from babies and small children as they are much more susceptible to the harmful radiation than adults. (While this is good advice, I feel that using a flip phone—or having no cell phone at all—would be preferable for one's health, while reducing the demand for so many cell towers.)

- **Be mindful of the second-hand radiation** from your own devices and those around you and how other people may be affected by the radiation from your techno-gadgets.

8 Trust me: I'm a doctor

I don't know what it is about medical buildings or doctors' offices, but they always seem to put me in a bad mood. (Even though I know that it's the effect of all the EMFs that make me feel so wretched, I always seem to forget this until after the fact, when the damage is done.) This time is no exception, although I could reasonably blame it on the fact that consulting a neurosurgeon has never been high on my list of fun things to do.

Dr A is reputed to be the best neurosurgeon in Vancouver. Like many of the highly skilled doctors in the city, he has a cool, clinically detached demeanour that his patients must find quite calming. I study him closely and am reassured to see that he doesn't bite his nails. This is good. Finding a neurosurgeon who is calm, steady and without any discernible neuroses is a good first step, although I have no intention of actually going *ahead* with surgery. After all, I teach others how to heal themselves so, obviously, I'm going to do the same. I just want to find out what my options are.

It's early June 2012, barely two years after my acoustic neuroma diagnosis in Ireland, and I'm sitting in the neurosurgeon's office with Lewis, to discuss my situation. There is also a young medical student who's taking notes before we even begin. Dr A asked if she could sit in on our conversation, and I agreed. Now, though, I'm not so sure. Sitting behind his desk and pointing at the MRI scan of my skull, his computer screen angled towards us, he begins by telling me I have an acoustic neuroma (also known as a schwannoma), which is a benign nerve-sheath tumour that, in this case, is growing on the eighth cranial nerve—known as the vestibular auditory nerve responsible for balance and hearing. I know all this as I've already done extensive research since being diagnosed, but then I realize that the lecture is for the benefit of his student.

I turn to her and ask her to kindly leave. It's nothing personal. I just want to be able to focus, and having so many people in the room is distracting me. It's bad enough having this kind of conversation with a complete stranger, without having another stranger clinically observing me as I ride an emotional rollercoaster from the pits of helplessness to the heights of fierce determination to fix this myself, and back again. Rollercoasters always make me sick.

Lewis looks at me as if I'm being uncharitable, and I telegraph him right back. *I refuse to be treated like a lab specimen—just another case study en route to her medical degree. What's wrong with these doctors? Don't they have an ounce of sensitivity or humanity in them? Can't they see how hard and scary this is? Can't YOU?* But it's a bit too much to telepathically transmit in under five seconds, and I don't think he quite got it all. Plus, I'm being unreasonable, as he *does* know how scary this is …I think.

Dr A is unperturbed. He resumes his discourse as if I'm perfectly sane and normal, and proceeds to tell me what my options are. This worries me— me seeming perfectly sane and normal when I no longer feel that way, and I am concerned that whatever decision I make in my current frame of mind might be the wrong one. My usual positivity and intuition seem to have gone out the window, crashing messily onto the street 11 storeys below and then running like crazy to catch the #99 to Commercial Drive, which seems to be the only kind of drive that counts. But I continue with the façade and pretend to be listening attentively, while The Voice inside my head tells me how things *really* are. *Don't kid yourself. You're incapable of healing this thing so just be thankful that there are alternatives.*

"We can operate to remove the tumour or do a series of radiation treatments," says Dr A. I feel so furious I want to punch something. I'm stunned by this explosive side of myself, which is completely out of character. Where is all this rage coming from? Some deeper, wiser part of me realizes that I'm angry at losing control—over my body and my life—and scared that this might forever be the case, despite what I believe about us all being capable of self-mastery and conscious evolution. But I'm also furious at the whole medical system. *How can doctors be allowed to irradiate you when that's what caused the problem in the first place?*

But could he be on to something? Perhaps I should get the radiation. He's a *neurosurgeon* so he must know what he's talking about, even though he's had no training in nutrition, hasn't researched the biological effects of EMR, and is clearly unaware that the body's symptoms are never random but the logical result of some environmental or other factor. Nonetheless, perhaps I should bow to the superior wisdom of this doctor—and then puke my guts up on the floor, sliding all over the neon-green radioactive toxic vomit as I ask myself (too late) how filling my body with carcinogenic radiation will eliminate a tumour caused by other, just as deadly, radiation on the outside. Thanks, anyway, but I think I'll pass.

Dr A has already asked me questions about cell phone use and which ear I hold the phone to. (My right, of course.) I know where he's going with these questions—and the kind of database into which my answers will be fed—yet he claims that no one knows what causes these growths.

"I know this was caused by microwave radiation," I tell him, "and lots of other people with neuromas say the same thing. Plus, there's scientific research confirming this, so I don't know why you say that no one knows the cause."

"There's not enough evidence to make that assumption," he says, and I want to strangle the man, sitting there denying what I know to be true about my body—not to mention all the scientific research that he clearly hasn't read. But I know that this is what medical doctors do; they tell you what's happening to you, and what you need to do about it, completely disregarding your direct experience, your body's natural healing abilities, and any wisdom or self-awareness you might have.

"So," he resumes, "we can do a rectro-sigmoid incision, here—" he points to the scan, indicating the base of the skull below my right ear, "and reach inside to scrape the tumour off the nerve." Gosh. He makes it sound so *easy*. "Or we can start with some radiation and see how that goes."

I'm incensed by this approach. But what I'm most angry about, I now realize, is that I may be forced to undergo surgery if I can't get rid of this tumour fast enough myself. My anger is fuelled by fear, of course, as I may not have any choice. It seems to be growing fast, so I don't have a lot of time to mess around. Yet, with my next steadying breath, I feel sure I can do this. I don't know if this fierce determination comes from my own desire to heal myself naturally, or to prove this doctor wrong. Either way, it's emotional fuel that I plan to put to good use.

"Think about it," Dr A is saying, "and let me know which option you'd prefer."

As if I only have those two to choose from, I think. *You'll probably have no choice at all,* The Voice chips in, *"and this thing won't go down without a fight. You think you can meditate it out of here? Ohhmmmm, no, I don't think so.*

Ignoring TV, I tell Dr A that radiation is *not* an option, just so he doesn't get his hopes up. I'm sure it's a lot less work than an eight-hour surgical intervention using tweezers and making delicate mini-moves while trying not to sneeze. Then it occurs to me that if he admitted that these tumours were caused by WiFi, cell phones etc, and if people realized the dangers and took preventative measures, he might be out of a job.

As my mind goes AWOL, I'm vaguely aware of Lewis asking him some questions, and of Dr A saying something about sending me a report so that I can make an informed decision. But I've already made my decision. I'm going to heal this myself.

9 Going under the knife

Never say never. Despite all my valiant attempts to heal myself over the past six months, here I am, in December 2012, contemplating my worst nightmare. It's the night before surgery and I'm numb with fear. The terror that grips my body is making me tremble all over and I try to joke about it so it backs off a bit and lets me breathe, and so that Lewis won't be crushed by the weight of my worry.

"I need this like a hole in the head," I tell him. "Let's call the whole thing off and go to Tahiti. I don't think they get tumours there, with all that lovely sunshine, fresh fish and sandy beaches."

"You'll be fine," he assures us both. "I'll be right there waiting for you when you come out and you'll bounce back from this faster than anyone else. You know how impatient you are, always wanting to be first."

He holds me tightly as we lie spooning in bed, and I know I won't sleep a wink. My mind is pre-living the surgery, imagining the saw cutting through my skull, bone dust flying everywhere... There's still time to cancel this, I tell myself. Maybe there's some other therapy that will work—something I discover if I just wait a little bit longer. But I know I've already waited too long and that too much damage has already been done. I'm almost deaf in my right ear and Dr A has told me I'll probably lose whatever hearing remains on that side, due to the surgery.

I'm furious with him for not operating sooner and saving my hearing on that side—but just as furious with myself for not being able to cure this on my own. How can this be? How can I teach empowerment and self-mastery and all the other stuff that seems to work so well for everyone else but hasn't worked for me? What kind of fraud am I? Have I just been talking the talk, all along, but not walking it?

"No, you haven't," Lewis tells me firmly when I express these concerns. "You've done everything possible to heal this yourself. You're amazing and you're being terribly hard on yourself."

Perhaps, I think. I've been so hell-bent on fixing this that I've lost touch with the spiritual side of me—the part I used to be so connected to that fuelled my intuition, before I began to feel so much physical agitation in my body. It will be another three years before I realize that the radiation has been agitating my nervous system all along, creating this ongoing internal fight-or-flight response and making it impossible for me to relax, heal or find any kind of peace. And, of course, for as long as I was still being exposed to the radiation that caused the tumour, recovering from it was impossible.

At 5am, the alarm goes off but I'm already halfway out of bed, all keyed up and wanting this to be over as soon as humanly possible. I'm so parched that my tongue is stuck to the roof of my mouth and I can hardly talk. Not being allowed any liquids for 12 hours before the surgery has meant that I haven't had my usual litre of water during the night. No matter how much I drink during the day, chronic dehydration has been another ongoing challenge—yet another symptom of radiation overload that I've blamed on other things.

When we arrive at the hospital, we have to wait to get checked in at the front desk. Lots of people going under the knife this morning, it seems. Finally, we're through and are directed to the surgical ward. Clutching Lewis as I go, I walk on shaky legs that no longer seem to bend at the knee, and my heart and soul seem to have gone off on a last-minute package holiday together, leaving my body hollowed out and empty.

We're ushered into a small green room with equipment crawling up the walls. I'm given a hospital gown, told to strip and to wash myself down with some disinfectant liquid that smells like drain cleaner. I proceed as directed, using as little of the caustic fluid as possible, opting for more of an aura clean than a toxic bodywash.

When I lie down on the gurney, the cold metal makes my skin retract as if I've been shrink-wrapped. My anxiety is spiking and my heels are knocking uncontrollably on the hard surface. A nurse comes in and I ask her for something to calm me down. I can't handle this, I tell her. I need something. She hands me two pink pills and a tiny cup of water. I guzzle it greedily, wishing she'd brought me more, and I ask if the drip can be set up ASAP.

Lewis takes hold of my ankle and I zoom in on him. He's trying so hard not to cry, and this must be the only thing he's ever failed at—unless, of course, he's not trying not to, in which case I love him even more for his huge heart. He's a solitary pillar of compassion in this room full of well-oiled machines. Two more come in, armed with a plastic gun and trailing wires. They grab hold of my head and start parting my hair. An overpowering smell of glue charges up my nose, almost knocking me out, and they proceed, without a word, to stick electrodes to my scalp. While I'm holding my breath and fighting to control a claustrophobic panic, someone grabs my arm and inserts the IV. I've never suffered physical abuse in my life, but this feels like a brutish assault. What would it cost for them to be gentle and to treat me like a human being? Is it because I haven't given them a tip? I imagine flinging them all away from me and transcending this torturous place, rising up through the ceiling, the electrodes fanning out behind me like small white kites in the wind. But Lewis has tethered me to the Earth and I hold on for dear life.

They wheel me out of the room, and the drugs seem to kick in just as Lewis is forced to let go, filling me with a calm detachment—or maybe just the exhaustion of defeat. They park me in an anteroom and a man in a white coat comes up to me, identifying himself as the anesthesiologist. He tells me to stick out my tongue and sticks out his own, in case I'm a bit dimwitted. I stare at him mutely, transfixed by the horror of it. His tongue is so ghastly that I'm concerned for his health—and mine. *This is the man responsible for keeping me safe during surgery?* His tongue has large black patches along the back, deep grooves along its length and a thick white coating that indicates a sugar addiction and bad diet. He repeats the order and I stick out my tongue, safe in the knowledge that he won't be as traumatized by mine as I am by his. If I were him, I'd get a tongue transplant ASAP and I certainly wouldn't be sticking it out for all the world to see. Surely there's a law against this kind of thing, especially for doctors…

…and then I'm gone.

10 Coming to a head

Five seconds later, I wake up. But my head is wrapped in a big bandage and I've got tubes coming from every limb and orifice, so it must have been a bit longer than that. Lewis is by my side, beaming love and eight hours' worth of relief at me through his tears.

"I did it!" I say, feeling euphoric and invincible. He hugs me tightly and seems to be at a loss for words. But I make up for it, rabbiting on about how easy it all was and that I really should do this more often. *I feel so good!*

Dr A comes in, wearing his usual serious demeanour. "The surgery was successful," he says, "and we were able to remove all of the tumour." Wait. Wasn't that the plan? Was there ever any doubt? Probably. But who cares? These drugs are *amazing*.

I thank him and tell him I'd give him a big hug if I weren't bound to the bed with all the tubes. He looks relieved. *Keep me on these drugs forever*, I tell him. Knowing how much I hate drugs, he smiles—I think. No, hang on. It's gone and he looks all serious again. I must have imagined it.

Accepting Lewis's grateful handshake on his way out, Dr A heads off to check on his other patients and I take in my new surroundings. I'm in the ICU ward in a private room, but I might as well be in a bus station. The traffic out in the hallway is almost as bad as on 4th Avenue—or maybe I'm just a bit sensitive after all the skull-drilling. Despite having been pumped full of anesthetic and other drugs over the past eight hours, I'm alert and wide awake. I feel happy to be alive, and I hope that's not due to the medication. I'd be really annoyed if I only wanted to live because of some drugs that were chemically altering my brain and giving me a false sense of happiness when, in fact, my natural state was one of cranky creativity and I was being kept in an artificial state of contentment, which never leads to any kind of angst-driven genius or disruptive extraordinariness and would be like having my soul anesthetized and permanently owned by the pharmaceutical industry. Yuck.

Lewis needs to go home for some rest and normalcy, so I settle down to observe the various forms of life in the Neurology ICU. I'm still figuring out some of the behavioural patterns when a nurse comes in with a tray of food.

This, of course, is fodder for further research and documentation. The items looks vaguely familiar: chicken (or is it fish?) in a state of advanced dehydration, a badly abused tomato, some elderly green peas, mashed potatoes (I think), and the universally renowned hospital cure for all diseases—jelly (aka Jell-o).

Wait! Hidden under the napkin, there's a little tangerine—an oasis of fresh, raw goodness, although it's probably from Peru and has been sprayed to death by poorly paid Peruvian workers who have pesticide poisoning but are too disenfranchised to sue their employers. *I must be more positive,* I tell myself. I can't heal if I'm so negative about everything (which is also a bit negative). I decide, therefore, that this little orange is probably from *California,* where it was born and raised in a sunny little orange grove tended by Earth-loving bohemians who would never dream of spraying anything nasty on their little citrus babies. I eat it and it's delicious. I can do this.

But then a nurse comes in with a little plastic cup and I know what's coming.

"Time for your medication," she says, handing me the little cup. There are two garishly coloured pills in it.

Drugs! All body systems go on red alert. (It's one thing to get drugs during life-saving surgery, but I think my body's had quite enough, thank you.) "What are these for?" I ask.

"The pink one is a steroid to prevent any swelling on the brain and the purple one is an antacid to counter the acid the steroid creates in the stomach."

"I never take antacids," I say. "They're very bad for the body. I don't want to take this."

"You have to take it," she says. "If you don't, having too much acid could damage the lining of the stomach."

"I don't want to take the other one, either," I say, my anxiety mounting.

"Those are the doctor's orders," she says with a shrug. "Maybe you should talk to him about it. But you really don't want to risk any swelling of the brain, honey. Not a good idea." She smiles as she leaves and I'm grateful for her warmth, which almost makes me cry. When did that simple human gesture become such a rare commodity in healthcare?

I stare at the pills, every part of me resisting them. I look up to make sure no one's watching, and I break the steroid pill into small bits. I knock back about a quarter of the pill with some water and then contemplate the antacid. Damn, I hate these things. I know how much harm they do and how many doctors prescribe them, when most people actually need *more* stomach acid. They don't realize that their symptoms are almost always caused by not having *enough* acid—and that they're similar to the symptoms you get when you have too much. Few medical doctors know this and would laugh at you if you tried to enlighten them.

After much angst, I swallow the antacid pill. Now I need to distract myself, so I settle back against the pillows to resume my observations of life around me. I've lost track of time but it must be early afternoon. In the next room, separated from mine by an opaque glass wall, another patient seems to be having a hard time, groaning incoherently every half-hour or so. I don't know if the groaning is due to recent surgery or if the surgery was supposed to get rid of the groaning. Either way, I feel sorry for him/her being in so much pain.

I'm thankful not to be in severe pain, although the right side of my head feels very tender. Yet it also feels numb, which is weird. I take a bite of chicken-fish and give it a good long chew. Maybe working the jaws will relieve some of the tension in my skull.

Suddenly, there's a strange feeling in my chest. It feels as if there's a big lump of dry clay stuck in my oesophagus and I'm finding it hard to swallow. The chicken-fish isn't going down properly. It seems to be stuck at the top of my stomach and it's as if my stomach has shut down. *No more deliveries. Sorry.* I immediately realize that it's the antacid. I knew it was not a good thing for me to take. I normally take *extra* hydrochloric acid with my food and I won't be taking any more of this stuff.

I call for the nurse, and the young woman who got me settled after surgery comes bouncing in, willing and eager to help. I explain to her what's happened and ask if it's possible to get some blended food from the kitchen. I can't seem to eat anything solid, since taking that pill, and it will be another two days before I can eat normally again.

She says she'll send a message to the kitchen, but it could be a while before I get anything. (Another 24 hours, as it turns out.)

In the meantime, I try to relax. I read a bit and take lots of deep breaths to try to nudge the chicken-fish into my stomach.

It's dark outside and the nurses seem to be changing shifts. The cheery day nurse pops her head in the door to say goodbye. She is petite with a big heart and the perfect disposition for calming frazzled nerves. She waves from the doorway and says she'll see me tomorrow.

Another young nurse, who's just come on duty, bounces into the room, introducing herself as June (Julie?) and telling me to call her if I need anything. I thank her and say I'm fine.

After lying there for a while, though, I start to feel uncomfortable. The top of the bed is up too high for sleeping but I can't lower it as the controls are down the outside of the bed and the IV stops me from reaching it. I ring the call bell and wait for the lovely June–Julie to come in.

Instead, an older nurse arrives. Her nametag says *Jasmine* and she seems annoyed to have been summoned.

"Could you please help me lower the top of the bed?" I ask. "And I'd love a softer pillow, if possible. This one is hurting my head."

She glares at me, adjusting the bed with a lot of noise and heavy sighing. "You can do this yourself," she says. "This is not a hotel!"

I'm too stunned to speak as she marches out of the room. No soft pillow for me, I guess.

I lie there, suddenly feeling vulnerable and depressed, as if the stress of the surgery is only now starting to catch up with me. I realize how alone I am. My parents and two sisters are in Ireland and I told them not to fly over for this, although they offered to. Taking care of them would mean more stress for Lewis and I don't want *them* to be stressed, either, seeing me like this. Most of my friends have fallen away, due to my radiation intolerance. No more meeting up in cafés (with free WiFi) or going to any social events (ditto). This makes me very *inconvenient*. As a result, I've become very isolated, preferring to be on my own rather than always having to ask friends to do me the massive favour of turning off their cell phone or meeting me at the beach or my home so I'm not exposed to all the radiation. Of the two good friends that remain, one is away on holiday and the other is at work.

I feel weepy, even though I tell myself it's probably just the effect of the drugs. My head is throbbing on the hard pillow, my neck aches and I'm starting to feel less-than-loving thoughts about Jasmine.

I press the call bell again and June–Julie comes in. I ask her if she could please send in her co-worker, Jasmine. I want to talk to her about the way she spoke to me earlier. After all, I've got nothing else to do, lying here immobilized in bed.

Jasmine finally arrives, two young nurses trailing behind her.

"You wanted to talk to me about something?" she says, sweetly.

I take a deep, calming breath …and then I take another one as the first one didn't work properly.

"It's my first night in intensive care," I begin, and it feels as if I'm telling them a bedside story, with the three of them standing there, rapt, waiting to hear what happens next. I'm thinking: *Shouldn't this be the other way around?* But that could just be the effect of the steroid I took earlier (although I stuffed most of it under the mattress where some bedbugs will someday ingest it and start doing the Macarena on the tiled floor). Even with that small amount, I've had psychedelic waking dreams for the past few hours, with visions of huge woollen knitted butterflies (knitted in a plain stitch), and underground carparks covered from floor to ceiling in multi-coloured plush carpeting, where oval-shaped futuristic cars swish by soundlessly, leaving thick grooves in the deep pile that sways slowly in their wake, like something from the movie *What Dreams May Come.*

"It's my *first* night in intensive care," I say again, "and I don't think it's unreasonable for me to ask for a softer pillow or for you to help me lower the head of the bed. The very nice—" (I almost said *much nicer*) "day-shift nurse told me to ask for whatever I needed and said she was there to make me as comfortable as possible."

Jasmine doesn't miss a beat. "I think it's important for you to learn how to take care of yourself as soon as possible," she says, and the two young nurses turn to look at her.

Does this woman have trouble with her eyesight as well as her capacity for compassion? This is the *intensive care* unit, after all, not a DIY centre.

"Jasmine," I say, with the supreme patience only possible in someone who's so medically tethered and cathetered that any truly satisfying drama-queen histrionics would cause me a lot more pain than this is worth, "since I have an IV in my left arm, a broken finger in my left hand—" (I broke it two weeks ago, making the bed, and I've told Lewis that doing any more housework is just *too darn risky*), "both legs are immobilized by these pneumatic pumps to prevent blood clots, I have a blood pressure monitor on my right thumb and my head feels a little tender because the surgeon sawed through my skull and then scraped around inside for eight hours or so, and I just thought that a little bit of help in lowering the head of the bed and perhaps bringing me a pillow that's not filled with rocks might enhance my physical and emotional well-being and justify your existence."

I'm not sure I actually said that last bit about justifying her existence out loud, but I think she got the general idea.

11 What's wrong with this picture?

With exquisite tenderness, Lewis lowers my head into the warm water, supporting my neck as he soaps my hair and washes away the surreal experience of the past four days in the ICU. I haven't slept at all for five days, which I attributed to the steroids, but I later realize that the high levels of WiFi and cell phone radiation in the hospital were probably largely responsible. Trying to recover from brain surgery for the removal of a tumour, while being bombarded by the very same microwave radiation now known to cause these tumours, is one of the many ironies that become apparent as I peel away the layers that cover up the deeper truth.

Where would I be without this man in my life? I lean on him in every way—as my closest friend, my partner, my emotional anchor, my chauffeur, my shopper, and the sole breadwinner until I can work again. He is carrying a heavy load for us both and I feel, again, the inherent wrongness of the situation. In just a couple of years, I've been catapulted from the relative youthfulness of my early 50s into the throes of old age. I hardly recognize myself in the mirror. I am haggard, worn out, wobbly and easily startled. My skin is thin and loose, perpetually dehydrated and stripped of its elasticity. Premature aging is one of the most devastating effects of electromagnetic radiation overload, stealing precious years of your life that you will never get back. While I once had the genetic advantage of looking young for my age, I've now gone the other way, closing the seven-year gap between Lewis and me and hurtling past him into my biological 80s.

Over the next few months, I battle with this vulnerability. My balance is shaky and I have to hold on to railings when I go up or down stairs. With zero hearing in my right ear, I can no longer tell where sounds are coming from or how far away they are, which is scarier and more destabilizing than I could ever have imagined. If I'm out walking and I hear a loud noise, I can't tell if it's a motorbike down the street or my stomach rumbling. I must do a 360° scan before crossing the road, and simple errands are a challenge in ongoing vigilance. With any background noise, it's hard to hear someone speaking to me. Worst of all, however, is the nerve-zapping inside my head. I thought the electrical buzzing would cease after surgery. Instead, it has been replaced by a persistent zapping on the nerve where the tumour used to be. I've gone from baby Taser to a more mature electrical jolt that's often painful. It seems to be triggered mostly by the ongoing dehydration, and I continue to drink at least a litre of water every night, with little effect. If I don't drink enough, though, the zapping speeds up, eventually becoming constant, like a small pneumatic drill inside my head.

So when (former) friends tell me that turning off the WiFi or cell phone is a hassle, or when I sense their reluctance to go out of their way to meet up in some low-EMF location, I reflect on the rather more significant and permanent hassle of having a brain tumour. I understand that they can't relate to what I'm feeling, but do they think I'm just looking for attention? Or am I just not worth the extra effort? Countless other distractions compete for their attention—meetings, Facebook conversations, morale-boosting Tweets, places to go, things to do, e-mails to answer, clients to cultivate, friends with no limitations. Having travelled the world and worked for prestigious international organizations, I'm used to being mobile, independent and self-sufficient, and I feel diminished by how much I must now apologize for: *I'm sorry I don't have the energy. I'm sorry I can't drive to your place. I'm sorry I can't go to that café. I'm sorry for the inconvenience.* In our wireless world of constant connection and instant accessibility, my sensitized system is like a digital dinosaur and I cannot compete.

The need for human connection is not being seen for what it is.

Thankfully, my brain still works fine, and what little energy I have I keep for the few clients I still work with. They, in turn, keep me sane, providing the opportunity for me to express to them what I most need to hear, and I love them in the unique way that comes from sharing the deepest truth of who we are. I'm grateful for their commitment and I feel honoured to still be a part of their journey, even as my own becomes more challenging, testing my wisdom and my own teachings like never before. Some part of me knows that there is a purpose to all this pain and that I will somehow figure out what it is.

In the meantime, I no longer have a life. It has been consumed by my debilitating neurological and physical symptoms, which distract me and keep me in a state of perpetual anxiety—about what's going on inside my head, about my future and my work, about my marriage and friendships, and about my ability to ever regain any kind of normal, productive, fulfilling existence. I try meditating but cannot relax. My body is agitated, unable to settle or focus on anything. I feel I'm trapped inside a perpetual loop of trauma, with all the symptoms of Post-Traumatic Stress Disorder. I try psychotherapy but it doesn't help. I send regular e-mails to Dr A, reporting my symptoms and asking him if they are normal. For the first few months, he says they are. After six months, however, he tells me that there must be something else going on. I should have fully recovered by now. There must be something in my environment that's causing the ongoing symptoms. I'm sure he's wrong and that there must be some re-growth of the tumour for me to be feeling like this. I cannot seem to shake the fear of my body somehow blindsiding me again, with something else beyond my control.

It's another year before I realize that I'm being exposed to high levels of microwave radiation (from WiFi and a cordless phone) from the apartment above us, where our landlady lives. But it's only when we go on holiday to Mexico for some relief from the crushing strain, that I realize what's been going on. As we check out the various available hotel rooms, trying to get as far away as possible from the WiFi at reception, I realize that I can physically feel which rooms are receiving a signal. We check this with a cell phone, noting which rooms get the most bars, and the hotel's technical officer joins us with his own device for checking signal strength, confirming what I've been feeling. A big piece of the puzzle suddenly falls into place.

After blaming my diet, my lifestyle, my constant worrying and the surgery itself, I realize that my ongoing exposure to microwave radiation has been causing almost all of my symptoms—and creating many new ones. The damaged nerve in my head has become a sensitive antenna that picks up all forms of electromagnetic radiation. I can tell from 10 metres away if someone has a cell phone turned on. I can feel the signal from a WiFi router. And I can tell when a digital electricity smart meter is transmitting one of the many high spikes of microwave radiation that it emits, day and night.

The damaged nerve has become my most reliable radiation meter, zapping me whenever I'm exposed to a strong electromagnetic field. Other symptoms—intense cranial compression, nervous agitation, jumpiness, tics, spasms, insomnia, headaches, stabbing pains and anxiety—confirm that I've found the true culprit, now that I understand how it affects the body. The more research I do into electromagnetic radiation, the more I discover about its insidious, invasive nature, the many biological effects of exposure and just how much scientific evidence there is (many thousands of independent scientific reports![19]) confirming the harm being caused. Finally, things are starting to make sense, and it's a huge relief to know that I'm not losing my mind or imagining things.

Yet this newfound awareness is like a double-edged sword. While it's reassuring to know what's been making me so ill, the rest of the world seems oblivious. Everyone around me is charging ahead with normal life, addicted to their wireless gadgets, and living their lives online with their smart phones stuck to their bodies like limpets. The more I learn, the more I recognize the dangers and the more isolated I become.

The world has no patience for this. Having free WiFi everywhere is so much fun that no one wants to be bothered by something that's not affecting them. Really, Olga, what *is* your problem?

Even Lewis sometimes finds my intolerance intolerable. When we go out for a walk, I ask him to please turn off his phone, which he carries in his pocket. He sighs with great forbearance and usually obliges, but he sometimes refuses to turn it off, saying he's expecting a call from a client. At those times, I feel abandoned and must dig deeply within myself to find compassion and understanding for him—as he has so often done for me. But I am angry that I have to ask—sometimes even plead—for him to protect my health. And I'm flabbergasted by the irony; back in the 90s, Lewis invented one of the very first devices for blocking radiation from cell phones.[20] Even though he was ultimately forced by the mobile-phone industry to cease and desist with his product (and was physically threatened, just in case he hadn't got the message), he is well aware of the dangers. Yet here he is, my one remaining beacon of sanity and support, nonetheless caught up in the collective frenzy of constant connectivity, convinced that it's essential for his business and for ensuring our financial security.

Yet the need for human connection, which is what actually drives this whole frenzy, is not being seen for what it is. It will be a long time before that happens …and even longer before people are willing to recognize or admit to the subconscious needs that drive them.

On those days when my man sides with the status quo, and I'm desperate for a healthy, sustainable way to reconnect with my world, I feel utterly alone. The greater my awareness of what's going on, the greater my despair at the widespread denial that it's a problem.

12 Delayed reactions and realizations

We're never given more than we can handle. Who made up that saying? Whoever he was, I want to set him straight. Yes, of *course* it was a man. Women know better than to spout such nonsense, knowing how many have died giving birth to *more than they could handle.* Unfortunately, they can't stick around long enough to go down in history as having said that *we're sometimes given more than we can handle.* But I don't have time to go off on tangents like this because I'm in the middle of something (our king-size bed), having a meltdown.

Sleepless nights, constant zapping in my head, dehydration that leaves my throat so dry I can't breathe, neck pain, cranial pressure, fears of my life being over, loss of my friends, social isolation, costly consultations with uninformed healthcare practitioners, dwindling resources and escalating symptoms with no end in sight… it is more than I can handle. My body is exhausted and I feel beaten. I want to find my OFF switch and check out. I'm a prisoner in my own home and even *that* isn't safe. Unable to get away from the ongoing exposure, I feel my tolerance decreasing while my symptoms get progressively worse—a common reality among those affected by EMR.

I'm having flashbacks as my mind retroactively makes sense of things that made no sense at all, at the time. The long-haul flight to a family wedding in Europe, which left me feeling so deathly ill that I could barely function. Relatives I hadn't seen for years were shocked by my appearance and my former husband was convinced I had cancer. (That was a crushing blow— wanting to look my best for him, having happily remarried, yet ending up looking worse than I ever had in my life.) I now know that it was the effect of all the radiation on the flight that made me so ill …but *he* didn't know that.

The one-night stopover in Amsterdam, en route back to Canada in 2011, when I didn't sleep at all in our rented downtown apartment. With over 25 full-strength WiFi signals coming at me from all sides, I now know why I couldn't switch off.

It's as if my brain is doing a rapid rewind, recapturing and collating all this previously unrecognized evidence, bringing it to my attention in one vast indigestible lump of retrospective revelations that make me cry even harder.

I'm a mess of conflicting emotions—rage at being lied to by government and the industry that has knowingly harmed me; grief at what I've unwittingly put my body through when it's trying so valiantly to keep me going; despair at not being heard or protected by my friends; regret at not discovering the truth sooner; self-blame for not being smarter, doing more research and knowing better; deep sadness for all my diligent, wasted efforts to heal myself; and more anger at all the compromises I made with friends and others, allowing myself to be exposed to more radiation, instead of standing my ground, saying no, and being assertive when it mattered most.

There's nothing like a good crying jag to make you feel alive, even if you sort of wish you weren't. Immersing yourself up to your eyeballs in self-pity is sometimes the only way to experience the true depth of your feelings. Letting it rip is far healthier than keeping it all trapped inside, festering and corroding your bits—as long as the only casualties are the hundreds of balled-up paper hankies littering the floor like cheap pompoms at a parade that no one came to watch.

That pathetic image makes me sit up straight and take stock of my sorry self. I breathe deeply to initiate some healthy recalibration and fling the last hanky into space, followed by two more balled-up unused ones because the forceful flinging felt so good. This is beneath me. I know better than to wallow in self-pity and defeat, given what I teach and believe in. I know that feeling disempowered is designed to get me to fight back, to assert myself, and to find a way to reclaim my autonomy and self-respect (while inevitably having a few meltdowns along the way). This is what I teach and know to be true: our challenges in life are designed to make us strong, once we understand what they represent and what we are being called upon to do. We're challenged to flex and make strong whatever emotional 'muscles' have been wobbly, due to whatever fears and insecurities we develop growing up. And we can only do this in the face of resistance, pushing back with whatever emotional resources and resilience it takes to reclaim our right to exist, grow and thrive.

So get a grip, I tell myself, *and stop being such a hanky-wasting wimp.* I need to be more of a ball-buster, although I can't really imagine myself in that role. It's not even a term I use, and I imagine myself only being capable of busting balls the size of jaw-breakers (those marble-sized hard sweets, known in Ireland as *gobstoppers*, that we used to buy as kids), rather than the much more daunting *testosterroneous* kind. I sense some strength and sanity trickling back into my poor exhausted bod and I take an objective mental inventory of all that I have lost.

My business has gone down the tubes. My health has hit rock-bottom. I'm 57-going-on-75. Most of my friends are busy being someone else's friends. My husband is over-worked and over-worried. I'll probably never see my parents again as the WiFi and other sources of radiation in airports and on airplanes makes it impossible for me to fly home. I've spent a fortune on EMF-shielding devices, bed canopies, fabrics and EMF meters. Our savings are becoming less and less worth saving. Because of the city-wide free WiFi, I can no longer access the healthcare services I need. I can't even go to the dentist—not that that's something I desperately *want* to do, but I don't want to end up a toothless old crone, either, slurping Complan and mumbling incoherently through loose lips and gummy gums. Our home is making me ill, and our landlady refuses to accommodate me in any way whatsoever, even at our expense and at no cost to her. This means that we will have to leave our home in Vancouver, and somehow, somewhere, find a safe, low-EMF place to live.

This last bit does the trick. I am now officially angry, revved up, raring to go and finally ready to *do* something.

My anger has cleared my head, and I'm starting to remember who I am, what I'm capable of, what I teach others to do when the going gets tough, and what it's all about. It's over three years since surgery, but only now do I start to fight back.

What the heck took me so long?

13 Learning the hard way

"I have a confession to make," I tell Lewis when he comes home one afternoon from a meeting downtown. "I ate the last four squares of chocolate, on my own, without you, all in one go, selfishly, greedily, while you were out, with no thought whatsoever for you, our marriage or anything else. I'm sorry. I just couldn't help myself."

"Well, I guess it's better than having the other kind of meltdown," he says, sitting down beside me and placing a bar of my favourite chocolate on the table in front of me.

"And they all lived happily ever after," I say, gleefully fondling my next fix. But I have another confession to make and it doesn't feel half as funny. "Sometimes this is the only thing that gets me out of bed in the morning," I say, holding up the bar of chocolate. "Isn't that pathetic?"

He looks at me sadly.

"There's you, too, of course," I hastily add—and it's true; Lewis is my anchor and my reason for persevering on those days when I don't feel like persevering.

But I'm aware that all my knowledge and hard-won wisdom go out the window when I'm so physically depleted that I have difficulty holding on to the deeper truth. Plus, I'm lonely. The absence of female friends who understand our irradiated reality leaves a gaping void. We women need our girlfriends! They're not just our emotional support system and our sounding boards; they're also a source of mood-boosting oxytocin, which kicks in when we connect and share from the heart.

Even though I have bouts of fierce determination to somehow resolve things, I can't seem to sustain a positive focus. Even *that* requires physical energy that I don't seem to have. The neurological symptoms have not let up since surgery, and the non-stop zapping, tingling, pressure and tension in my skull is exhausting. No one can explain the ongoing issues and I sometimes even doubt that the radiation is the problem.

But I know that it *is* and, if I start doubting this reality, I remind myself of the huge social pressure to fit in, to do what everyone else is doing, to go along with the status quo and to not make a fuss. Hey, it worked for cigarette companies. Of course, it's working for the wireless industry, too.

Yet, due to my isolation and emptiness, I'm gaining insights that I might not otherwise have gained. Being so disconnected from friends, social events and work-related interactions, I become a detached, objective observer, watching from a distance as life goes on in a frenzy of non-stop wireless connectivity. In being physically disconnected from that world, I see just how disconnected we have become in all the ways that matter.

Family members no longer talk to each other at mealtimes, preferring instead to text their friends or read the news on their iPad. People out walking their dogs barely register the changing seasons, the people around them, or even where they're going, so focused are they on their cell phone. Everyone on public transit has their head down, eyes glued to their phone, existing in a virtual vacuum.

Young mothers with their babies in a body sling hold their phone right against the infant's body—and then put it in the sling, with the phone not even a centimetre away from the tiny body. They are unaware of even the simplest precautions they can take—or that precautionary messages can be found deeply hidden in the settings of their own devices. The minimum distance recommended by cell phone manufacturers is often difficult to find on their devices but varies from about 5mm to 10mm ...for adults. People dining together in restaurants spend most of their time on their phone, updating their virtual friends on their fascinating choice of dessert, rather than enjoying the company of the actual living, breathing person in front of them.

Young people have become so addicted to their wireless gadgets that they often get hysterical if they lose them or if their phones get confiscated by their parents. And their dependence has as much to do with a physical necessity as an emotional need for significance, relevance, importance and a sense of belonging and connection.

My hearing loss prevents me from orientating myself properly, creating a kind of *echo dislocation*. But it's not just me; I may be more aware of it because I've been *forced* to be, but we've all lost our bearings, surrendering so many of our mental and emotional faculties to a digital device.

We no longer look at maps or rely on our own sense of direction to find our way around; instead, we use GPS and allow a disembodied voice to direct us. We rarely exercise our brains by making mathematical calculations, instead using calculators on our wireless devices to add up even the simplest of sums. The cultural enrichment of learning a foreign language has been reduced to a quick online translation. We go online to find a partner, having lost the art of communicating and connecting with others face to face, in honest, heartfelt ways. We fill out online questionnaires to determine our most likely perfect mate, and we spend hours in virtual engagement versus true in-person intimacy.

We have apps that correct our spelling, and most young people have never learned proper grammar or punctuation. We've lost the art of using rich and powerful language to convey our deeper feelings, instead relying on emojis and replacing our linguistic aptitude with a virtual '*apptitude*'. We use apps to help us sleep, to monitor our heart rate, to tell us when to water our plants, to create background white noise, to let others track our location, and to provide entertainment for our pets. There are even wireless sensors to tell parents when their baby's nappy (aka a diaper) needs to be changed. Instead of doing this the time-honoured, hands-on way, parents can now insert *a wireless radiation device*—right next to the delicate organs of their vulnerable child, whose DNA may be irreversibly damaged by the radiation—to save them the insufferable inconvenience of having to peek inside the nappy. Of course, babies have their own very smart way of alerting parents to their needs—*crying*—but who wants to be bothered with something so emotionally messy when a wireless gadget can remotely do the job for you?

In hospitals, healthcare centres and doctors' offices, wireless devices are running the show. Prescriptions are dictated into a wireless laptop and printed out on a wireless printer at reception. Patient histories are recorded on iPads as you sit immersed in a sea of radiation known to create and/or exacerbate almost every one of the symptoms that patients are there to address.

I've appealed to doctors, asking them to kindly turn off the WiFi in their office, since it creates so many health problems. Yet they all refuse to do so, claiming that it's *inconvenient* and that they couldn't manage without it as all their systems are now wireless. But you can hard-wire your computers, I say; you can get corded phones, and you can ask people to switch off their cell phones, just as they are now told they can't smoke …can't you? Nope. Apparently not.

One Vancouver-based doctor, who specializes in anti-aging medicine, fails to see the supreme irony of having microwave radiation in his office—radiation that's known to prematurely age the body by destroying its protective antioxidants, and inhibiting production of the sleep hormone melatonin, which also protects the body against cancer, among other things. Hang on a sec, though. Maybe I'm not cynical enough. Maybe he *does* know how harmful it is and is very cannily ensuring a perpetual stream of patients desperately and forever dependent on him to stop their unstoppable accelerated aging. But is he smart enough to realize that it's aging *him*, too? Or has the radiation already affected his cognitive function to the point where he's forgotten his duty as a doctor (you know, one of those people who take an oath to *do no harm*)?

I'm bewildered by the insanity of it all—and the denial. When microwave ovens became a popular convenience in the late 1980s, by which time almost

50% of homes had one, it wasn't long before health-conscious West Coast Canadians decried the damage that these irradiating devices were known to do. Yet here we are, less than two decades later, up to our eyeballs in microwave radiation as if it's suddenly perfectly harmless and benign. Maybe most people are too young—or too uninformed—to know that microwaves were (and still are) used as military weapons. In my research, I discovered that the British Government targeted certain Northern Ireland communities during the IRA troubles, hitting them with microwave radiation so that they became sick and less able to fight back. And there are several other examples of this radiation being used by governments to intentionally cause harm.[21]

With its reputation for being a peace-loving, humanitarian country, Canada has always seemed to be a safe place. I begin to realize that I've been terribly naïve. I know little about politics, but quite a lot about human dynamics—which usually tells me all I need to know about people, no matter who they are. I know that there are dodgy politicians and that all kinds of shady deals are made with major industry players, but I've tended to trust that the Canadian Government is not causing too much damage. Having grown up in a family with strong opinions, I'm aware of a desire to be right, which I've tempered a lot (well, maybe just a *little*), but I really, *really* wish I could be right about this—that the government knows better than to knowingly harm its own citizens by bombarding them with harmful radiation. Unfortunately for me and for millions of others, I turn out to be horribly wrong. The government is not looking out for our interests and there is far more nefarious stuff going on behind the scenes than we're aware of.

Now, as I observe the rapid proliferation of WiFi and cell phone towers all around me, I wonder how I can have meaningful connections with people who are so emotionally, physically and logistically committed to their wireless devices. How can I even begin to connect with them when the radiation disconnects me from myself and scrambles my brain, making me dizzy, dense and disoriented? Failing that, how do I find joy and connection in my isolation?

If I can't stay in meaningful contact with others, I can at least stay in touch with myself, and so I do the only thing I can do to hold on to me and to make this whole sorry mess seem worthwhile.

I write another book.

14 Making things write

My writing fills my days, expanding my inner world as my imagination transports me far away from the reality I want to escape. My brain seems to be on fire, sometimes churning out so many ideas that I spend all night scribbling indecipherable notes like some demented scientist. There are times that I feel so much cranial pressure and tingling, it's as if there's a whole army of ants on nano-trampolines inside my head. At other times, it feels as if there's a metal claw clamped to my right ear. With so much nerve-zapping, insomnia, pain, pressure and neurological agitation, I wonder if I'm losing my mind, but then I tell myself that truly insane people never question their sanity. Right? Am I right?

I nonetheless manage to write, self-publish and print two complete books in less than a year. I don't care if anyone reads them (although it might be nice to know that they've helped someone or made them smile). But they're really for me, giving purpose and tangibility to the morphing madness around me.

The first one is non-fiction, based on my work.[22] *The Alphabet of Powerful Existence* is a series of 52 themes, in alphabetical order, with two for each letter of the alphabet (such as acceptance + authenticity, boundaries + balance, connection + community …you get the idea). There's one for each week of the year, designed to boost well-being, wisdom and worthiness in simple, practical, everyday ways. Each theme has a definition, followed by bullet points on why it's important, why it's difficult to practise, and how you can embody it in your life. It's a sort of quick download of a lot of the concepts I teach and strive to live by. I need to remind myself of this stuff and why it's important. I need all the reminding I can get, given how I'm feeling about things. As soon as I get that out of the way, though, my mind seems to kick into a completely different gear, dispensing with the real world and conjuring up an alternative reality filled with the *strangest* characters.

This second book (*A Talk on the Wild Side—imaginary interviews with unlikely sources of wisdom*)[23] is packed full of fiendish fun and creative deviance, and it practically writes itself—whether I like it or not. It grabs hold of me and won't let go until it's done. I'm just the transcriber, frantically trying to keep up with the non-stop stream of information that comes at me from every conceivable source. All kinds of inanimate objects start talking to me. (Yes, I know; I'm still questioning my sanity, too.) I have intense conversations with a toilet, a parking metre, a peanut, a strawberry, a park bench, a fly, a hub cap, a hyena, a maple leaf and even a fossilized *T. rex*. *They* talk to *me*. I don't seek them out. They arrive in my head, unbidden, and keep pestering me till I strike up a conversation. They are persistent, loud and impossible to ignore and it's a lot easier to talk to them than to tune them out. The funny thing is that, when I do, they all have unique messages to share—the kind of profound wisdom that I never expected to find in such normally silent, passive places (not that I expected to find anything there at all). I learn a lot from these imaginary oracles, which seem to show up just when I need to hear what they've got to say.

T. rex is one of my favourites. This one is big on humour and small on pleasantries, setting me straight on my misguided notion that humans are the most advanced, intelligent species and that the dinosaurs died out because, well, they were never going to fit in with our modern way of life (regardless of the fact that they were wiped out by asteroids). I had no idea that dinosaurs had no memory—did you? They lived purely by instinct, with no memories of past negative experiences cramping their style or deflecting them from their purpose ...*unlike humans*. I never really thought about how much our memories shape or distort our lives. Yes, of course, it's useful to remember what harmed you, so you don't go back for more abusive treatment from your ex-partner or eat more of that cake that had you pinging off the walls from the sugar blast, and it's wonderful to have a store of positive, feel-good memories to relish as you grow old and reflect on your life. But many of our early negative memories pull us off track, diminishing our self-worth, making us fearful of risk, and preventing us from living life to the max.

Many of the other interviews make me laugh out loud, which is good for my soul and a welcome reprieve from the seriousness of survival. Daunted by all the radiation, I know how *deadly serious* life can become and I have to keep reminding myself that *it's just life*, and that none of us gets out of here alive. We might as well give it all we've got and live as creatively and as powerfully as we can. So I resolve to stop being so *careful* about things and to have as much fun as possible, despite the challenges. *If it isn't fun*, I decide, *I don't want to do it*—and that's when all these oddballs come out of the woodwork. When it comes to creativity, we all have our own unique voice and mode of expression; figuring out what that is and sharing it with our world is part of the magic of being human. If we don't dare to share, we'll never know what kind of impact we could have had, or how much fun.

The interview with the toilet is another one of my favourites. Each interview has its own theme, and this one is all about denial and disowning our 'stuff', which seems appropriate, right now. We all have some of that (no point in denying it), particularly in terms of what goes on inside our bodies. *Out of sight, out of mind* is how we tend to think of what goes in and, even more so, what comes *out*. How many of us want to know or care where all our human waste goes? Who gives a shit, right? I know, I know; it's not my favourite topic, either, but the toilet's take on things is surprisingly insightful and funny.

Several others are clamouring to be interviewed, but I already have more than enough for this first book. There's a light bulb, which keeps harping on about its illuminating insights into what we *think* we see yet fail to see, even when it's right in front of us. There's an old wooden boomerang in our garage, and (you guessed it) it just *keeps* coming back, pestering me for an interview, no matter how many times I say NO! That's what *I'm* doing in my life, it tells me—going around and around in circles and getting nowhere. The theme of this one is *interpreting life's signs*, it seems, and it keeps taunting me, saying I'm resisting its insights, and that *some* people just don't *want* to move forward, because they're in denial and they want to *stay* there. I finally relent, just in case I'm missing out on some nugget of wisdom that proves absolutely vital to my existence. (FYI, it does offer *one* interesting insight.)

Then there's my toaster, which gets cranky when anyone tries to stuff big fat bagels into it or use starchy white bread (not me) that burns within minutes and then they whack the thing, trying to remove all the broken burnt bits. The toaster claims that everyone has their own 'smoke point'—the point at which they flip and lose it—and it explains why it's helpful for people to have their triggers activated. But it says there are *two* sides to this story and it won't be drawn out until I'm willing to sit down with it and do a proper interview. What the heck? Do *you* get this kind of flack from your toaster?

In the meantime, the book is doing its job—distracting me from myself and reminding me that life is full of cosmic surprises, simple wisdom and the kind of magical connections you least expect to make when you feel disconnected from almost everything.

PART 2
FIGHTING FOR OUR LIVES

15 Seeking safety ...in all the wrong places

My condition is getting steadily worse. I can no longer remain in our kitchen for more than 20 minutes as the cranial pressure and pain caused by the WiFi radiation from the apartment above us is too intense for me to tolerate. Since Lewis is working for both of us, I want to at least do the cooking and prepare our meals. I become a master at healthy fast food, whipping up tasty dishes in 15 minutes or less. But then I have to scurry downstairs to try to recover from the effects.

We decide to buy another RF-shielding canopy to put over our dining-room table, so that I can sit and eat in comfort. We already have one for our bed, which helps a little with sleep, but it doesn't block the strong electromagnetic fields coming from the wiring, which is affecting me more and more. Our costs are mounting as my capacity to work diminishes. With ongoing exposure, my tolerance is going down and my symptoms are getting worse—which is typical of this condition. As is the case for so many others affected by wireless radiation, I'm learning as I go—and learning most things the hard way, through personal experience.

But I'm also reading and researching as much as I can, and a document is taking shape without my consciously intending it to. There is so much information, so much scientific evidence of EMR-related harm, and so many people out there sharing their stories that it's overwhelming. The vast body of material is matched only by the government disregard, deception and denial, with the wireless industry doing all it can to create public doubt and confusion. Not that they need to try very hard, with everyone so addicted to their wireless gadgets and mobile lifestyle. In just a few short years, we've become a society that expects everything to be fast and free—free software, free apps, free WiFi access, free connectivity—all delivered at the speed of light, which is how fast this microwave radiation travels. It also behaves like light, radiating out in all directions from multiple overlapping sources (WiFi routers, cell towers etc), while being amplified by the signals coming from the countless wireless devices themselves.

Sometimes I wake up and wonder if it's all been a terrible, crazy dream. How can this be happening? What kind of insanity has taken hold of us that we're bombarding ourselves and our planet with the very same microwave radiation that's been known since the 1950s to cause 'radiowave sickness' and has been used (and is *still* being used) as a military weapon? What happened to intelligent life on Earth? And those of us having what science confirms is a *biologically correct reaction* to this harmful radiation are dismissed as flakes. *What? You've got a problem with this fabulous free stuff floating through the air, making life so much easier?* Yes, and some of us have trouble tolerating arsenic, too. Silly, I know, but there you go.

No matter how much research or reading I do, I will never be able to cover it all. New studies are being published almost daily and new websites and blogs are being created by those with a compelling story to tell and data to share. But the more I read, the more motivated I become—and the more incensed. It's not that I'm horribly angry and on the warpath for all those nasty people out there making my life hell. It's more a case of seeing through the many deep layers of dysfunction that prevent most of us from realizing what's really going on, until we're forced to. *I've* been forced to and I know I'm also being forced to fight back, to reclaim my right to live and to find my own unique way of powerfully expressing that.

Easy to say, but how the heck do I do it? Charity begins at home, they say, and so does homework—the kind you need to do to assert yourself and stand your ground in a healthy way. We're having an unpleasant time with our landlady, who has turned very negative and unfriendly towards us. Now she doesn't even say hello, and we know she illegally entered our home while we were away. She wants us gone and very clearly harbours a grudge against us for having dared to stand up to her on a few occasions.

But I've got more important things to think about, such as where we're going to live. Where can we go to get away from the pervasive and ever-increasing microwave radiation? Even in the tiny fishing villages of Mexico, with primitive houses and unpaved roads, cell phone towers provide phone service for everyone—and every café has WiFi. Lewis tells me that caves can be quite warm and cozy, once you get a good fire going, but I think I'd find them a bit gloomy. Then there's the option of camping out in the wilderness, but where would I go to buy chocolate? We could go deep into the interior of BC and find a spot where no cell towers are allowed, but how long would that *last*, with wireless installations spreading across the planet like a virus? We'd probably end up all crusty and hillbillyish, wearing Wellies all year round, wrapping ourselves in crocheted shawls, trudging to the outhouse in three feet of snow, and bathing once a month.

We decide on an interim approach and find a place to rent on Vancouver Island between two small towns and (according to the online antenna-finder) far enough away from cell towers to probably be okay—for now. The thought of leaving my favourite city doesn't fill me with joy, but I know I have to go. I won't last much longer if I stay, and having access to the beach and all the other wonderful amenities within a few blocks of home just isn't the same if you're six feet under.

By the end of May, I've finished my document and it has turned into a 25-page report addressed to Vancouver's Mayor Gregor Robertson, as well as Prime Minister Justin Trudeau, local MPs and some of the media. A blend of my personal story, the facts about microwave radiation, the symptoms of electro-sensitivity, a large sample of the scientific evidence confirming harm, and some pointed questions for the government to answer regarding the escalating, unmonitored and unquantifiable levels of radiation around us, I'm hoping it will at least generate some kind of reaction. In mid-June, I finally click *send*, launching *No Safe Place*[24] into the ethers.

16 A crisis of epidemic proportions: the evidence

Once upon a time... the Earth was flat. Smoking was good for you. Thalidomide was great for morning sickness. Asbestos made for excellent insulation. Nuclear power was the way to go. GMO crops were a godsend to farmers everywhere. And hydrogenated oils were a cost-effective choice. Now, we have WiFi and mobile networks, connecting us with everyone, everywhere, every second of every day... and creating a pervasive, virtually inescapable, unprecedented, unchecked, uncontrolled and rapidly escalating proliferation of radiation in our environment. But don't worry: the wireless telecommunications industry and your friendly health-conscious government say it's safe![25]

Like so many of those ill-founded claims, WiFi is now being promoted as a safe and beneficial technology in industry-sponsored studies and PR. Consequently, the media have featured many misleading, inaccurate and incomplete reports about WiFi radiation, claiming that there is no apparent causal relationship and that there is zero evidence supporting the experiences of those with EHS.[26] Such claims merely reveal the reporters' ignorance of the latest research—and perhaps their own addictive love affair with their cell phone. Some have claimed that reactions to electromagnetic radiation are psychosomatic, which is an insult to the countless individuals who had no idea that EMR was causing their ill-health and only discovered the very clear causal relationship after years of research, functional impairment, huge expense and misdiagnosis.

Nonetheless, such theories are likely to be very reassuring to those who are unaware of the facts and to the many others who really don't want to know about the dangers.

Instantly penetrating cement, metal, plastic, clothing, cars, bone, muscles, tissue and skin, radio-frequency/microwave radiation affects us all, all the time, within minutes of being exposed.

Evidence of harmful effects: quick facts*

• There is now **10 billion times more radiation** in our environment than there was in the 1960s.

• In 2006, scientists estimated that, if current trends continued, **50% of the population** in Austria, England, Ireland, Germany, Sweden and the state of California would be feeling the effects of electromagnetic radiation by 2017 (see http://bit.ly/2CmsBLM). Canada would be no different.

• Swisscom, the Swiss telecommunications company, says non-thermal wireless radiation **"has a genotoxic effect"**, causing **"clear damage to hereditary material [DNA]"** and an **"increased cancer risk"**.

• Insurance companies, such as Lloyds of London, now refuse to provide coverage for health-related damages resulting from the radiation from wireless devices.[27]

• **EMR adversely affects the blood cells of ALL individuals**, whether they feel the effects or not.

• **EMR damages cell membranes**, causing them to **leak calcium** and create many health issues, such as **altered brain function, autism, infertility, electromagnetic hypersensitivity, hypocalcaemia, DNA damage, thyroid problems, osteoporosis, endocrine imbalances, early dementia, asthma, neurological disorders and multiple chemical sensitivities.**

• **Autism in children is doubling every five years**, paralleling the rise of EMR, and there is now a **1-in-50 chance** of a child developing or being born with autism in North America.

• **Almost every grade in every elementary school** in North America has **at least one child with autism**—a disorder that was nearly unheard of a generation ago (see http://usat.ly/NZXM1i).

• Electromagnetic radiation **breaks down the all-important blood–brain barrier**, causing leakage of toxins into the brain and the death of neurons, which can result in **early dementia** and **Alzheimer's disease**.

• Just 5 minutes of exposure to microwave radiation from WiFi can cause **cell mutation, oxidation and rouleaux**—all of which are associated with **illness and disease**.

• The average cumulative whole-body exposure from a smart meter at a distance of 3 feet is about 100 times more than that from a cell phone (see https://goo.gl/Po9e6K, at minute 2.17).

* This information is taken from my No Safe Place document. See elsewhere in this chapter and in the document itself (https://olgasheean.com/no-safe-place/) for additional references to the studies/data mentioned.

While the physical effects of electromagnetic radiation are numerous and widely reported, the effects on mental health have received less attention. They are no less real, however, and no less disturbing.

Are we losing our minds?

German psychiatrist Dr Christine Aschermann reports an "increased occurrence of cognitive and psychological disorders with exposure to telecommunications".[28] Personality disorders, short-term memory loss, inability to concentrate, amnesic aphasia (difficulty finding words) and parapraxia (carrying out inappropriate actions), as well as irritability, mood swings, physical weakness, sleep disturbances, chronic exhaustion, agitation and lack of motivation are other common symptoms that she has seen as a result of radiation exposure from the increasing use of wireless devices. There is also a loss of ethical values, empathy and sound judgement, as well as an increase in aggression and violence.

An increase in suicides has also been linked to wireless radiation, says Aschermann. "[In 2009], it was reported that a great number of France Telecom employees had committed suicide. Recently, the electronics firm Foxconn in China was affected by 10 suicides during the first five months of the year. Following the introduction of TETRA into the Israeli army, a series of young conscripted soldiers self-harmed. At the Siemens office in Munich, where the DECT telephone was developed years ago, there were reports of people committing suicide by falling from a height."

Furthermore, she says: "We know from the research carried out since the 1950s by the Russian and US American military that specific moods can be evoked and manipulated. Thus, depressive states, fear, mania, pain, lack of motivation, and hallucinations are possible responses, depending on the frequency, wave-forms and other characteristics of the radiation."

Scientific fact versus political spin and misinformation

It's no wonder that most people are confused, ambivalent or dismissive of the dangers of EMFs, given the vast amount of political spin and misinformation promoted by the telecoms industry and industry-friendly governments … not to mention the complete lack of public-awareness campaigns. Below are some of the claims that governments and industry-funded scientists have made in an attempt to convince consumers that they need not worry about adverse health effects and can continue to enjoy their wireless devices …while supporting the multi-billion-dollar industry and the governments that benefit from billions of dollars in licensing fees every year.

SPIN: Non-ionizing (microwave) radiation does not generate enough heat to do damage and, therefore, this non-thermal form of radiation is not harmful to humans.

FACT: Scientific studies—and the telecommunications industry itself— confirm that non-thermal radiation *is* harmful to the human body.[29]

- "Weak non-ionizing electromagnetic radiation in the environment can be linked to more 'modern illnesses' than even the pessimists thought possible," says Dr Andrew Goldsworthy. "Modern science can now begin to explain how." It is not a heating effect, he explains, but an electrical effect on the fine structure of the delicate electrically charged cell membranes upon which all living cells depend. (See http://bit.ly/1taEDi3.)

- The American Academy of Environmental Medicine reports that: "Epidemiological studies demonstrate that **significant harmful biological effects** occur from nonthermal RF exposure" (http://bit.ly/24XtIpS).

- A **Swisscom patent** application clearly states that **non-thermal wireless radiation "has a genotoxic effect** [...] elicited via a non-thermal pathway" and that "when human blood cells are irradiated with electromagnetic fields, clear **damage to hereditary material [DNA]** has been demonstrated [with] indications of an **increased cancer risk**." The international patent (See http://bit.ly/1OQbG4V), filed in 2003, was for technology to reduce the 'electrosmog' from wireless local networks, intended to reduce the cancer risks associated with non-thermal exposure to microwave radiation. (For more details, See http://bit.ly/1BCVa0W.)

- **A British epidemiological study (confirmed by Swedish, Japanese and Italian findings) shows an association between long-term use of**

a cell phone and acoustic neuromas (See http://microwavenews.com/uk-study-points-acoustic-neuroma). Although acoustic neuromas (which grow on the eighth cranial/auditory nerve) are 'benign', rather than malignant, they can still kill you.

SPIN: Extremely low frequency (ELF) radiation has no significant health effects.

FACT: The electromagnetic fields that are most harmful to humans are those in the ELF range and also the radio frequencies that are pulsed or amplitude-modulated by ELF (see http://bit.ly/1PlASJZ for the following three points).

- ELF radiation has been scientifically proven to **damage cell membranes**, causing them to leak calcium and create many health issues, such as **altered brain function, autism, infertility, EHS, hypocalcaemia, DNA damage, early dementia, asthma and multiple chemical sensitivities.**

- Electromagnetic radiation can damage the **all-important blood–brain barrier**, causing leakage of toxins into the brain and the death of neurons, which can result in **early dementia** and **Alzheimer's disease.**

- Gland cells are particularly sensitive to radiation, which can **damage the thyroid and endocrine system, disrupting the metabolism**. Even short-term exposure to radiation from a cell phone tower has been shown to **increase cortisol levels**, with long-term exposure resulting in **permanently elevated adrenaline.**

- EMFs disrupt the production of melatonin, the body's only antioxidant, resulting in high levels of damaging **free radicals/oxidative stress and accelerated aging.**[30]

- Inward calcium leakage in the neurons of the brain stimulates hyperactivity and makes the brain less able to concentrate on tasks, resulting in **attention deficit hyperactivity disorder (ADHD).**[31]

"The time to deal with the harmful biological and health effects is long overdue. We must reduce exposure by establishing more protective guidelines."[32]

SPIN: There is no demonstrable medical proof of harm being caused by WiFi or smart meters.

FACT: The damaging effects of microwave radiation from cell phones, WiFi and smart meters can now be medically demonstrated.

- The damage done to red blood cells from brief exposure to RF radiation can be seen via live-blood-cell (dark-field microscopy) analysis, which reveals cell mutation, **oxidation and rouleaux** (aggregation of red blood cells) (see https://youtube/y4JDEspdx58).

- Just 5 minutes of exposure to WiFi radiation results in cellular damage associated with **pathological processes** (See https://vimeo.com/100623585, at minute 4.48).

- According to the *BioInitiative Report*,[33] bioeffects occur within minutes and at very low levels of exposure to EMFs and RF radiation—similar to those from cell and cordless phone use, as well as exposure to mobile phone masts (cell towers), WiFi and wireless utility smart meters that produce whole-body exposure. Chronic base-station-level exposures have also been shown to result in illness (http://bit.ly/1Xn4ZIV).

SPIN: Only vulnerable, hypersensitive or weak individuals are affected.

FACT: The damaging effects of EMR have been medically proven to occur in every human body.

- Dr Erica Mallery-Blythe, a former accident-and-emergency doctor now specializing in EHS, says these **effects occur even in those not experiencing symptoms,** and many of us may be electro-hypersensitive and not realize it. "Everybody has the potential to become electro-hypersensitive," she says, "[since] **every cell in our body, in our brain or nervous system is dependent on electrical signals**" (See http://www.dailymail.co.uk/femail/article-2331369).

- Many other doctors (such as Dr Dietrich Klinghardt[34] and Dr Andrew Goldsworthy) confirm that **EMR affects the blood cells of all individuals,** ultimately damaging their nervous systems, brains, reproductive organs and physical health.

SPIN: The supposed effects of EMR are intangible and cannot be objectively measured.

FACT: Medical doctors and researchers have identified biomarkers of EMF intolerance—biological indicators of EMR damage, found in everyone suffering from EMF sensitivity, as well as in those who had no idea that such a thing existed or that it could be making them ill.

- Exposure has been found to have a **damaging impact on melatonin, serotonin, dopamine, adrenaline, cortisol, testosterone, progesterone, T3 and T4 thyroid hormones and plasma ACTH** (which regulates cortisol) (see http://bit.ly/1rXJUcC and http://www.magdahavas.com/), among many others.

- Dr Dietrich Klinghardt[35] tests for particular biomarkers in those affected by EMF pollution: an **increase in inflammation markers** (TGF-Beta 1, MMP-9 and copper, which shows chronic inflammation, **hormone abnormalization and neurotransmitter abnormalization**) (see http://bit.ly/1Sc8I8G).

- Other medical tests for detecting EMF effects include live-blood-cell analysis, brain and nervous system analysis, and cardiac analysis (see https://www.emfanalysis.com/ehsbiomarkers/).

SPIN: When those with EHS were asked to detect the presence of cell phone radiation, from behind a curtain or closed door, they often couldn't tell when the radiation was present, or they reacted even though the cell phone hadn't been switched on—which proves that it's all in their heads.

FACT: This approach has since been invalidated, for several reasons. Many individuals with EHS can physically feel RF/microwave radiation, although they often don't know that that's what they're feeling. Even those who feel nothing, however, are still being affected at the cellular level.

- Most people feel nothing, since the effect occurs at the cellular level, beyond their conscious awareness. Only in those with sensitized nervous systems, or those for whom the strength/duration of exposure has created physical symptoms, will the effects be felt.

- To claim that people react physically to the mere suggestion of EMF exposure merely reveals an **ignorance**—not just **of how EMFs affect the**

human body at the cellular level, but of human nature itself. If you have a fear of spiders, heights or small spaces, and you're told that you might be given a tarantula, placed on a cliff or locked in a closet, you would instinctively experience anxiety, sweating and other physiological stress responses, whether those threats materialized or not. Yet the danger posed by EMR is very real and a fear of it is well founded.

- As Dr Mallery-Blythe points out: "Electromagnetic hypersensitivity is a **physiological issue, not a psychological one** [and] it can be seen as either a sickness or a supersense, depending on the environment of the individual, although it is essentially both" (see https://vimeo.com/100623585).

- French oncologist Dr Dominique Belpomme concurs: "**We know with certainty that electromagnetic hypersensitivity is not psychosomatic.**"

SPIN: Service-providers claim that WiFi/cell phone/smart meter radiation is safe, and the media haven't reported anything conclusive, so there's no need to worry.

FACT: Thousands of scientific studies attest to the damage caused by RF/ microwave and other forms of electromagnetic radiation.

- The results of many of these studies have been published in reputable medical and scientific journals such as *The Lancet, the International Journal of Neuroscience, the Journal of Applied Sciences Research, Electromagnetic Biology and Medicine* and *NeuroToxicology*, among others (see www.emf-portal.org and http://bit.ly/2EXRH0Q).

- Studies find adverse biological effects from WiFi frequencies (2.4 or 5GHz), with exposures of <16V/m (such as those from a WiFi-enabled device): http://bit.ly/1jsIPUp.

- **A $25m study by the National Toxicology Program of the NIH found that cell phone radio frequency radiation caused two types of tumours: glioma and schwannoma (acoustic neuromas).**[36] Twenty years ago, these tumours were rare. Now, they are increasingly common.

- "EMFs provoke major effects in the brain," says oncologist Dr Dominique Belpomme. "The most important of these is the opening of the blood–brain barrier. This allows mercury, organochlorines and other pollutants to enter the brain, where they cause various neurodegenerative diseases."[37]

- While some reports in the media claim that EMR doesn't harm us, doctors and specialists around the world are quietly helping those whose lives have been torn apart by the very real and devastating phenomenon of electromagnetic hypersensitivity. For a timeline of growing awareness of/landmark rulings regarding EHS, See http://www.emfwise.com/awareness.php.

Is this getting on your nerves?

The incidence of chronic neurological illnesses is rapidly increasing, with autism in children *doubling every five years*, according to Dr Dietrich Klinghardt.[38] And he knows why. "The only thing that parallels the exponential increase in chronic neurological illness is the increased exposure to manmade electromagnetic fields—largely in the high-frequency range from cell phone radiation, the Tetra network [...] smart meters..." With credentials, expertise and medical specializations too extensive to list, Dr Klinghardt is a recognized authority on EHS and the many diseases (ALS, Parkinson's, MS, autism etc) exploding out of control, due to the widespread proliferation of radiation. He has identified the biomarkers of EHS, adding considerably to the research carried out over the past 80 years—most of it showing biological damage being done by EMR. "As a scientist, you don't have to look very far," he says.[39]

Dr Martha Herbert, PhD, MD[40] is an expert in neuro-developmental disorders—particularly autism spectrum disorders (ASD). She has published papers in brain-imaging research, physiological abnormalities in ASD, and environmental influences on neuro-developmental disorders such as autism as well as on brain development and function. She also carried out a review literature on the potential link between ASD and electromagnetic fields (EMFs) and radiofrequency radiation, and found such an extensive body of literature that she ended up producing a 60-page paper with over 550 citations.[41] There are now thousands of scientific, peer-reviewed papers on the adverse health and neurological impacts of EMFs. Children are more vulnerable than adults, and those with neuro-developmental disabilities are even more so.

Although current wireless technologies were designed and promulgated without taking into account biological non-thermal impacts, we now know that significant adverse effects occur without the heating of tissue. "The claim from WiFi proponents that the only concern is thermal impacts is now definitively outdated scientifically," says Dr Herbert, whose findings are confirmed by thousands of scientists worldwide.

The evidence is now so vast and compelling that it would be hard for any diligent researcher not to be daunted by the sheer volume of data. Wireless telecoms service-providers and politicians who ignore this crucial evidence do a huge disservice to humanity, often vilifying, patronizing and insulting those with EHS, who are the early indicators that something is seriously wrong. With government health agencies turning a blind eye to the proven adverse biological effects, consumers tend to do the same ...unless they have personally experienced the effects of the radiation, done their own research and realized what a massive cover-up is underway.

17 Getting litigious

I have had several exchanges with our landlady, asking her if she could please turn off her WiFi when she's out during the day. She's gone from about 7.30am till late afternoon, and all she has to do is unplug her router when she leaves. But that's too inconvenient, she says. I then offer a practical solution—giving her a box lined with RF-shielding material in which she can place her router. This will prevent strong signals from radiating downwards into our living space but won't stop them from radiating outwards into hers. It's an easy, win-win solution, at no cost to her. After I practically beg her to try it, she finally takes the box, but then we hear nothing for three days. There's no reduction in the radiation coming into our home and not a word from her. I send her an e-mail to see if she's using it and I offer to drop in to check that it's installed properly. No response, but the box appears back on our doorstep the next day, with a Post-it note saying, *No, thanks.*

As I said, not a great deal of compassion or caring going on here—and, sadly, zero awareness of how wireless radiation damages everyone, whether they feel it or not, as well as plants and animals. Even though I tell our landlady that she has a legal obligation to accommodate a tenant with a disability. (Electro-sensitivity is recognized as a disability by the Canadian Human Rights Commission, yet she refuses to do anything to reduce the harm being caused to me—not even for the last few weeks of our tenancy. As I continue to experience stabbing pains, inflammation, dizziness, cranial pressure and tension, rushing from one shielding canopy to another to try to avoid the radiation, the situation strikes me as utterly insane. *For this, we are paying thousands of dollars in rent every month?*

I feel drained, ill and frustrated. Nothing I do or say makes a difference. Despite us having been model tenants, our landlady cannot find it within herself to do the right thing. I am tired of being treated this way and I am angry. So I decide to take her to court.

I file a complaint with the BC Human Rights Tribunal, after being assured that they handle this kind of thing and that I can probably get legal assistance from their partner, the BC Human Rights Clinic. Yet even as I make these enquiries, I know I may end up regretting this move, as it feels toxic and negative to get into a legal battle. But I've had enough! Even if I lose the case, at least I'll have taken some action to stand up for myself and will feel better for having done that, even if no one else does.

Only when we move to Vancouver Island do I discover a vast online community, populated with people from all walks of life who have come together through a common cause: they have all either been directly affected by the invasive man-made electromagnetic radiation in our lives or have a loved one who was, and they are united in their efforts to make things right. *There were so many of them!* How could I not have known about all these people like me? I had felt isolated in Vancouver, believing myself to be in a very tiny minority—but only because I hadn't reached out and connected with all these existing online networks. I personally knew of only two other people who were being affected: a doctor who was getting migraines from cell phone radiation, and a woman who had been so incapacitated by EMFs that she had been bedridden for years. She had almost her entire house wallpapered in shielding fabric (which must have cost her a fortune). Other than that, I was alone in my electro-sensitive world.

And then I wasn't.

18 New place, same old scenario?

Moving from Vancouver to Vancouver Island by ferry (less than a two-hour crossing) turns out to be more exhausting than moving overseas, which we've done several times. After helping the movers pack our stuff and after organizing cleaners to help us clean the apartment before we leave, I know I'll have to contend with strong WiFi on the ferry. I'm already depleted and run-down from the ongoing exposure to EMR in our home, with little resilience for dealing with any kind of stress, so I'm not in ideal shape for this. We miss the ferry we had hoped to take at noon and sit for two hours in the queue, already wishing the day was over. I refrain from thinking bad thoughts about our landlady, knowing that this is a positive move and that things will very soon get better. I remind myself also that living there was toxic on many levels (all four storeys, in fact!) and that it's far healthier for us, emotionally as well as physically, to move to a cleaner environment.

Finally, I think, we'll be able to relax. Having checked the EMF levels in the house when we came to view it, we knew that there were some issues with the electrical wiring but felt confident we could fix that easily enough. We also thought we'd be able to buffer the smart meter, which was on the other side of our living-room wall, so I was looking forward to very soon having a healthy home environment. Sadly, this turns out not to be the case. I'm aware of the same horribly familiar buzzing and zapping in my head, accompanied by the usual compression and dizziness. When I take out my meter to check the electromagnetic radiation, I discover that we are, indeed, getting radiation from WiFi and smart meters from all sides. How could I have missed this? I realize that I must not have waited long enough when I tested the radiation levels the first time. When I leave my RF meter switched on, about 20 feet away from the smart meter, I see that the levels are spiking every 10–15 minutes or so, with a big spike occurring every 30 minutes.

We enter a bad patch. Lewis and I are spent—mentally and physically exhausted and so depressed by this new reality that we can barely function or be civil to each other. We nonetheless make an effort to restrain ourselves, knowing we're on shaky ground and that we need to be very gentle with ourselves and each other. I don't want to unpack. I don't want to stay but we have nowhere else to go. I find myself cycling down into despair and wondering where I packed those sleeping pills—not so I can get some sleep but so I can go on a one-way trip to a place where I'll never be bothered by radiation again. I seriously contemplate this. I'm not the suicidal type and I'm normally the first to jump in with some rallying positivity and practical suggestions for resolving a problem or crisis. But this one has bested me, while worsening me in ways I never could have imagined. From some remote place, I observe the person I've become and I seem pitiful. But I can't seem to muster the energy to care.

Later, I discover that microwave radiation often changes a person's personality, as well as mood, judgement, cognitive function and many other things. I barely recognize the person I've become, but it's not so much that my personality has changed; it's that my capacity to be my true self has been undermined by all the stress, immune depletion and rapid degeneration. It takes energy to be fully switched on and I feel as if I've been running on empty for a long time. Plus, I can no longer make the kind of choices or commitments I'd normally make, which changes how I show up in the world and how others perceive me.

If I didn't have Lewis, I couldn't do this. I could not manage without him, and I think of the other electro-sensitive individuals who don't have a partner to help them—or, even worse, had a partner who left because he/she couldn't handle the stress. Losing your health, normal life, livelihood, friends etc *and* your partner must be intolerable.

Lewis and I slowly regain some energy and our survival instincts kick in. After walking around like zombies for a few days, we take stock of what needs to be done. We throw everything we've got at the smart meter, covering it with the usual wire-mesh cage recommended for shielding radiofrequency fields and putting up several layers of shielding fabric on the inside wall behind it. Still, the radiation comes in, although slightly less strongly than before.

Our friend Marcus recommends covering the sides of the house with the same wire mesh, so Lewis heads off to the hardware store to buy several big rolls of the stuff. He spends the next few days tacking the mesh to the ends of the house—a one-storey rancher about 20 feet away from our neighbours on either side. All this manly stuff is good preparation for his Canadian citizenship application, and it starts to pay off. Once the mesh is up on both sides, the levels of microwave radiation go down.

We heave a massive sigh of relief. But then I start to get strange nerve-jumping sensations in both legs when I'm sitting or standing in certain places. I discover that the electrical fields generated by the wiring in the house are now affecting me—and maybe always did, without me realizing it. I haven't even begun to bounce back from the past five years of intense stress and this feels like another huge challenge. In my research, I discover that many people experience this same progressive intolerance—often first becoming sensitive to some strong electromagnetic field, such as the microwave radiation from WiFi or a newly installed smart meter, and then becoming sensitive to electrical and magnetic fields as their body is weakened by the ongoing exposure. The more exposure, the lower the tolerance and the less resilience the body has. Not a nice cycle to get stuck in.

But help is on the way, it seems, through some kind of cosmic serendipity. When Lewis returns from the local Saturday market, he tells me he met an electro-sensitive woman there who knows of a building biologist in the next village—a woman who has trained in assessing electromagnetic radiation in homes and offers practical solutions for reducing exposure and creating a healthier environment (similar to what Jim Waugh did for us in Vancouver, but more extensive). I get her number and arrange for her to come by. Even as I do so, however, something feels off. It's as if I'm heading down a path I'm not meant to be on. While I'm aware that I must find some practical solutions to the EMFs that are making normal life difficult, I also sense that there's a more powerful approach that I'm meant to be pursuing. For now, though, I must do whatever I can to give my body some relief so it can recover.

19 Expanding awareness

Annette Koch arrives heavily laden with books and all kinds of EMR-testing equipment. She's in the process of completing her certification in building biology and electromagnetic radiation assessment, and her head is swimming with information. It's an intensive course, requiring a knowledge of electricity and electrical wiring as well as of the various forms of electromagnetic radiation from wireless devices. She is also studying geopathic stress, dirty electricity, mould and other aspects of modern living that often create mysterious illnesses and conditions that doctors fail to diagnose.

She spends about four hours going through our house, testing the levels of electromagnetic radiation from our smart meter, our neighbours' WiFi and smart meters, our electrical wiring and our appliances. It confirms much of what I had already figured out with my basic meter, while adding a few more elements that end up making a huge difference. Our friend Marcus and his electro-sensitive wife Benita had already helped us greatly in identifying some basic culprits—such as the transformers that come with certain appliances, and the CFL bulbs that are supposed to be eco-friendly but actually emit high levels of harmful radiation. We had removed all these and now used only incandescent bulbs. The wiring in certain electrical circuits is faulty, Annette tells us, although it might not be considered as such by an electrician. It's not that electricians don't care about wiring errors, she says, but that they are oblivious to the biological effects of these EMFs.

"The majority of electrical errors are actually NEC (National Electric Code) violations" says Annette. "We get a lot of sloppy wiring and the code needs to be followed. We need government regulations around this energy. That doesn't mean we will have no fields. Electrical fields envelop us because plastic-jacketed wiring does not contain these fields. It would be much better if we all used metal-clad wiring, as this would prevent the fields from permeating our living spaces." Nonetheless, she says, with proper wiring practices, we can greatly reduce both electrical and magnetic fields.

Some of the wiring in our home is emitting high levels of EMR that are increasing my body voltage—something I hadn't considered and didn't have the equipment to test.

In my office, the levels are particularly high—around 4,000 millivolts—and they were also high in the bedroom. Annette explains that the levels in the bedroom, particularly, should be no more than around 10 millivolts in order for the body to achieve a deeply restful state and for it to heal and restore while sleeping. Guidelines from the Institute of Building Biology & Sustainability[42] (a recognized authority and training facility in electromagnetic radiation assessments) suggest that below 10 millivolts would be of no concern; 10–100 millivolts would present a slight concern; and higher levels would present a more significant concern. Nowadays, says Annette, it is hard to bring personal environments below 10mV, but most people find that they sleep much better if the levels are under 100mV.

The immune system cannot recover if the body voltage remains high throughout the night, she explains, and lowering the levels is essential for healing and recovery. With much running back and forth between the bedroom and the electrical panel, which happens to be in our living-room, she figures out which breakers need to be turned off at night so that restful, restorative sleep can occur.

This, combined with the shielding canopy over our bed, makes a huge difference. Sleep is deeper, less fragmented and more peaceful, although the zapping and dehydration persist. Using her various meters, Annette also figures out that it's best for me to work on my solid-state laptop using only battery power, while keeping it plugged into the socket, but with the breaker off. This way, I get the grounding effect of having the laptop plugged into the ground, which further reduces the voltage coming at me. The opposite proves to be true for Lewis, who uses a Mac computer, which has far higher levels of EMFs than my laptop. For him, the voltage goes down a little if he works on his laptop with the cable plugged into a live socket. But I can feel that the levels in his office, with the Mac, printer, backup drive and other appliances, are far too high for me and I avoid going in there.

At the end of the day, I'm exhausted. The process of assessing the electromagnetic fields in our home environment is intense, but I feel relieved to have discovered some other factors that were preventing me from recovering. Now, I think, I can start the healing process.

20 Electrifying facts

I delved deeper into the effects of electrical fields when I connected with Arthur Firstenberg—a tireless activist in the field of electromagnetic radiation and hypersensitivity, and founder of the Cellular Phone Task Force[43] in 1996. I first spoke to Arthur when I was working on a script for a video addressed to Prime Minister Justin Trudeau, and I wanted to interview him. But then this book leap-frogged over it, demanding to be tackled first. Some books are like that—pushy, demanding and fickle, with their own agenda, timeframe and attitude, haranguing you with their urgent messages, dragging you along for days without sleep, and then leaving you hanging with nothing to say for a whole week.

"Electricity is toxic to humans," Arthur told me. At some deep level, my body already knew this, but the fact had never really registered in my brain. Why would it *want* to? Electricity is such a fundamental part of our lives that I can't imagine trying to live without it.

Arthur started out as a mathematician and then went on to medical school in 1978, but he was unable to complete his studies due to illness, which he attributes to electromagnetic hypersensitivity brought on by getting over 40 diagnostic dental x-rays. In 1997, he published his first book, *Microwaving Our Planet: The Environmental Impact of the Wireless Revolution,* and I had heard that he was working on a second one, about the history of electricity. In a telephone chat in late 2016, he told me he had almost finished writing the book, entitled *The Invisible Rainbow: A History of Electricity and Life.* Published in mid-2017, the book received rave reviews from scientists, researchers, doctors and electro-sensitive individuals alike.

I spoke to Arthur again a few months after the publication of his book, which documents the development of electrical technology from 1746 to today, explaining how the evolving technologies have affected us. "We have an internal electrical system," he says, "and we live in an environmental electrical system. The book describes them both and how they interact. Electrical technology—particularly wireless technology—interferes with both our internal circuitry and the circuitry of the entire Earth. The amount of pollution that is already out there, and the pollution to be added in the next several years, is so intense that the only solution is to stop it. There's no escape from it any more. The only way to preserve life on the planet is to put a halt to it."

This is the key purpose of Arthur's book—to make it clear that we cannot ignore the reality and that we cannot continue like this. "I'm following in the footsteps of Rachel Carson," he says. "She put pesticides on the map; I'm putting electricity on the map as an environmental factor."[44]

> "Electricity is at once the spark of life
> and the undoing of it."
> —Arthur Firstenberg

While there are some things you can do to protect your body, Arthur says, they pale in comparison to the assault. You can shield yourself, to a certain extent, wear protective clothing, bathe in clay water that will absorb some of the radiation, or live in a part of the world where the impact is less serious. Arthur has chosen this last option to try to minimize his exposure, living in Santa Fe—an area where the conductivity of the earth is very high and therefore helps to ground the radiation. "You can do all these things," he says, "but the assault is becoming so tremendous that none of these options will work for very long."

Must we give up electricity in order to be healthy? In the long term, he feels that we must. However, that's unlikely to happen for quite some time. But are there things we can do to make electrical distribution safer? "Absolutely," Arthur says. "We can adopt a five-wire system of electrical distribution. This means having three hot wires, a neutral return wire and an isolated ground wire. The ground wire is still connected to the earth, for safety, but the neutral is totally isolated and carries all of the unbalanced current back to the transformer and the utility provider. This dramatically reduces stray voltage."

Given my very limited knowledge of electricity, I don't quite follow this, since I assumed that ground wires were connected to the earth for natural grounding. Not so, Arthur tells me. "Earth acts as the zero-volt reference for all electrical systems in most of the world, which ground all of the wiring to the earth, everywhere, and that means that the earth is constantly filled with ground currents from the electrical grid. When we're walking on the earth, then, we're vibrating at 50 or 60 hertz of alternating current (AC) [as opposed to the Earth's natural direct current (DC)—the Schumann resonance (7.83Hz)—to which our bodies are entrained], because the earth is full of these electrical currents. However, it is possible to construct an electrical system that does not do that."

So we can make electricity a great deal safer. However, says Arthur, "We cannot make wireless technology safer. There's no such thing. If you're broadcasting it deliberately through the air, it's going to have an effect, and it's going to be a disastrous effect."

If we look at the use of energy from a long-term perspective, Arthur says, in the way that native Indians consider our effects on the next seven generations, as a measure of sustainability, the industrial revolution itself is not sustainable. Each person is using too much energy and has too big of a footprint on the Earth. "Electricity is secondary to that," he says, "but if we really want a sustainable society, we have to develop technology a heck of a lot more carefully than we have been doing for the past few centuries."

I ask Arthur if he thinks being exposed to too much electricity could have caused my loss of hearing. "Hearing loss is usually due to either loud noises or microwave radiation," he says.[45] "So using WiFi, when you didn't yet understand the dangers, could have started the process. And the only thing I know of that helps with this is acupuncture."

I've tried this approach, working with many different practitioners, over the years, but it hasn't helped, even though I know it has helped many others. However, as Arthur reminds me, it's essential to find a practitioner who does not have WiFi or other sources of microwave radiation in their treatment rooms …which is now rarely the case. In the same way that I was unwittingly exposed to wireless radiation when recovering from brain surgery in hospital (not that I had any choice about this), I was almost certainly exposed to this same radiation when I went for acupuncture treatments in Vancouver.

Given Arthur's early exposure to high levels of radiation, I'm curious to know how he is coping now. "I've been in despair since my trip to Canada in 1990," he tells me. "I went from the Queen Charlotte Islands up to Alaska and then to White Horse in the Yukon and, the further north I went, the more per capita use of technology there was. In the far north, people have private airplanes, snowmobiles, motor boats and everything, and the imprint of the average Yukoner is greater than the imprint of the average American. That's what sent me into despair—the fact that I could not escape civilization. It not only followed me everywhere but, the more remote the location, the more intensely people were using technology to keep out the wilderness."

After that trip, Arthur went into retreat for six years and then all the cell towers starting going up. At that point, in 1996, he became a refugee, constantly on the run from the radiation and living in his car for several years, until he found his current home in 2009. Now, he says, he's hanging on to it with everything he has. It took him a total of 20 years to write his book— partly because he was unable to work for many years, due to the impact of radiation on his health.

"Had you finished it in 2000, as you hoped, it would not have covered so much invaluable material," I point out.

"That's true," he says, "although it also means that we don't have a lot of time left to fix this. And I'm far less optimistic now than I was back then. In 2000, you could still get away from it. Now, you can't. All my illusions are pretty much gone and I'm just facing the stark reality of what's happening to our planet and trying to do my part to stop it."

Arthur has done a great deal to expose the dangers and to explain the evolution of harm due to our increasing dependence on electrical and electronic devices.[46] Hopefully, his book will help raise awareness so that people start calling for safer electrical distribution systems and safe alternatives to wireless technologies.

Despite the compelling evidence, I don't think any of us want to give up electricity. We've never known life without it, but its effects on people have been known for over a century. In the late 1800s, Nikola Tesla is thought to have been the first person to experience what later became known as electromagnetic hypersensitivity. An inventor and a visionary in the fields of electrical engineering and electronics, Tesla has been dubbed the 'father of electrical engineering', and his intense experiences and explorations into electromagnetic phenomena seemed to be paralleled by an expansion of his psychic awareness. According to Cyril Smith, author of *Electromagnetic Man*, these phenomena included premonitions and the visualization of certain events in his life. "Tesla's hypersensitive experiences must have helped his intuitive appreciation of the invisible electrical forces," says Smith, "which he did so much to harness, and with such success." This makes sense to me, since being sensitive in one area often leads to sensitivity in another, and those who are emotionally sensitive and aware often tend to be more readily affected by electromagnetic fields.

But sensitivity to and tolerance of EMR have their limits and many of us are now at the tipping point, bearing a cumulative load of electrical charge that's pushing many of us over the edge. We can handle a certain amount, but if we keep increasing the dose, we inevitably reach a point of saturation and overwhelm when we can no longer withstand the harm being done to our bodies.

So the question is this: how bad do things have to get before we acknowledge the reality and create a demand for healthy, sustainable forms of telecommunication?

21 The immunological impact of microwave radiation

According to Professor Trevor Marshall, Director of the Autoimmunity Foundation in California, and a Fellow of the European Association for Predictive, Preventive and Personalised Medicine in Brussels, there has been an exponential rise in chronic disease since the 1950s, when VHF and microwave transmissions began. "The statistics show that damage to human immune systems has been continuous and incremental during that time," Trevor tells me. He estimates that maybe 10% of the population is already suffering the damaging effects of 4G and WiFi radiation, yet doctors and scientists are failing to recognize this because of the sheer diversity of illnesses that it's causing.

"Today, 60% of adults in the US are taking medication for some diagnosable chronic condition," he says, "and many of the rest, without a diagnosis, have learnt to live with a state of poor health, unexplained aches and pains, fatigue, and loss of concentration." There are other factors, he explains, but immune dysfunction from 50 years of exposure to microwave radiation is already exacting its toll. Mankind evolved without any significant natural sources of microwave radiation; since new forms of man-made radiation emerged in the 1950s, our bodies have struggled to cope with their effects. "Any level of microwave radiation affects human biology," Trevor says, "not just the stronger signal sources."

I ask Trevor about the proposed roll-out of the new 5G wireless technology, and he makes it very clear that it's extremely bad news for humans everywhere. "It involves millimetre waves (extremely high frequencies) producing photons of much greater energy even than 4G and WiFi," he says. "These 5G frequencies are known to have a profound effect on the human body. Allowing this technology to be used without proving its safety is reckless in the extreme, as the millimetre waves can directly affect all parts of the human body.

"People are being told that microwave and millimetre radiation has no effect on the human body at low levels. But there is a profound effect, and it has been documented since its discovery during the Cold War. Millimetre radars were causing major problems on both sides of the Iron Curtain, and many studies were performed to find out why. Then, in the early 1980s, the FDA was relieved of its responsibilities for electromagnetic health, and the conferences supported by its Bureau of Radiological Health were stopped. That is why the early literature is so important in coming to an understanding of the effects of high- and low-energy microwaves on the human body. For example, a large conference on Biologic Effects of Nonionizing Radiation was held in February 1974. However, the FDA, which provided financial support for publication of the 1974 conference papers, no longer has any research interest in non-ionizing radiation."

A CIA document, de-classified and approved for release in mid-2012, spells out some of the adverse biological effects of microwave radiation on the liver, spleen, lungs, kidneys, heart and DNA, among other things.[47]

Trevor explains that engineers only measure the radiation until it falls to 1% of its peak value, which can be easily read on their signal meters. "But the electromagnetic waves are bioactive down to levels of 0.0001%," he says. "Scientists stop measuring the signal long before it loses its bioactive potential. The lower energies penetrate deep into the brain—particularly a child's brain, since its skull is smaller than an adult's.

"As the frequency increases, each wave photon has more energy and a greater effect on the molecules it hits, but higher frequency waves don't penetrate as deeply because their energy is being transferred more rapidly into the tissues. So which is worse: more bioactive photons being deposited in just half of the brain, or fewer losing their energy deeper into the brain? Neither option seems viable to me. "

He goes on to explain why there is so much uncertainty, confusion and debate between the EHS community, government agencies and the industry (in addition to the vested interests of the latter).

"The EHS community will never win against industry until it stops arguing in terms of the units of measure that the industry has historically forced upon us. Those units have no utility other than to reinforce the fiction of SAR (specific absorption rate) being relevant to health. It is not, and it has never been proven to be. Correlation is not causation. Watts/square metre and its subunits continue to be emphasized (over volts-per-metre and decibel-milliwatts (dBm)[48]) so as to focus attention on heating, and to detract from the importance of the huge dynamic range in amplitudes of electromagnetic radiation in our environment."

And the idea that the effects of millimetre waves are confined to the skin only came about because engineers stopped measuring at far too high a signal level. "Our research has demonstrated that people with immune disease can reliably sense levels of as low a power as 110dB below the cell phone signal (which is 0.0000000001%, in layman's terms). I therefore believe we already have a huge problem on our hands, even before the addition of 5G technologies to our environment."

Trevor explains that no wideband meter can measure the lowest signals that the body can sense (which can be 300 times lower than most simple meters would measure). Biological harm therefore cannot be accurately measured with any test instrument that you can easily buy. "It takes an experienced operator and an expensive cumbersome instrument to measure signals at the -90dBm levels at which we have shown the body can produce a reaction," Trevor says.

"Studies have only taken place between about -37dBm and +50dBm, so researchers have only considered signals 100,000 times higher than what biology can reliably sense. The effect of low-level radio-frequency radiation has been ignored. No wonder the results of 'challenge' studies are usually 'inconclusive'. This is why our discovery that humans with immune disease can reliably sense levels around -90dBm is so important."

As with other 'safety standards' that were only debunked after years of pressure and mounting evidence (such as with the tobacco and asbestos industries), all this confusion plays into the hands of the profit-driven wireless industry …for the time being.

Based on 40 years of experience with clinical research, Trevor has developed an immune-boosting protocol that is helping many with EHS, among others. An increasing number of his associates are flourishing as a result of adopting his protocol and creating a low-EMF environment. They wear shielded clothing during the day and sleep in a good Faraday cage (a real one, filtering most dirty electricity and AM as well as other radio frequencies). Sound, restorative sleep is the key, he says. Their ability to deal with the electromagnetic environment has also steadily increased as they recovered. "Focus on that word: RECOVERY," Trevor says. "It is something that has vanished from modern medicine, which is preoccupied with treating symptoms. Back when I was trained in clinical research, it was our only goal. It is still my sole goal and, with the new knowledge from the past decade, I know it is now achievable." (For more information on his research, see his many PubMed papers, the study site: www.marshallprotocol.com, or his colleagues' knowledge base at https://mpkb.org/.)

The increasing radiation in our environment is nonetheless extremely bad for our health and must be addressed. Trevor suggests that all radio broadcasting (AM, FM and TV) could be replaced with landline and satellite, which would make the outdoor signal strength much more controllable (due to the great distance from the satellite). Indoors, we need wired technologies, and possibly LiFi (if it turns out to be safe). Google's balloons also offer a controllable signal environment, he says, if improved and properly implemented.

22 Fodder for our fears? 5G and the Internet of Things

[This section was kindly contributed by Kate Kheel*]

The worldwide rush towards 5G (fifth-generation) wireless roll-out is set to raise pulsing electromagnetic pollution to alarming new levels in order to increase available bandwidth, enable faster downloading of multi-stream videos and support smart meter/smart grid connectivity.

Realizing that digital human-to-human connectivity is saturated, and hoping to ensure continued innovation and future profits, the wireless telecom industry, along with governments and others hoping to share in the bounty, also decided to wirelessly connect all 'things' to the Internet—and dubbed it the *Internet of Things* (IoT).

The technology and bandwidth we currently use for 2G, 3G and 4G are not enough to support IoT, which will be used for applications such as driverless cars, artificial intelligence, robots, smart cities, virtual reality, augmented reality, augmented humans, and other tech innovations. So the telecom industry is in a mad rush to acquire as much bandwidth and wireless real estate rights and sites as they possibly can for 5G wireless technology.

Industry is predicting 50 billion connected devices by 2020, with the employment of escalating transmission frequencies. Although 5G will use many of the same frequencies used in cell phones and other wireless platforms, it will also use the higher millimetre wave frequencies (mmW), never before used for wireless telecommunications. Although mmW frequencies are able to carry vast amounts of data, they don't travel well through most building materials. Millimetre and centimetre frequencies such as 15GHz, 28GHz, 39GHz and 60GHz are expected to be put into widespread usage. These short-range, high-speed signals would require antennae to be situated around towns and cities at intervals of approximately 200–250 meters. For 5G to work, then, all of us would have to accept 'small' cells and their attendant infrastructure on lampposts and utility poles throughout our communities, outside our homes and, potentially, even inside.

Not only that, but Boeing and SpaceX, among others, have plans to launch thousands of satellites to provide broadband Internet globally. (Astronomers say that these radio waves will create light pollution, which will affect their ability to observe lower energy phenomena in our universe, such as the cosmic microwave background—a form of radiation left over from the Big Bang.[49])

So-called *smart* things are set to permeate every aspect of our lives. All things, machines and appliances are being upgraded and reconfigured to be smart. Untold new IoT applications and platforms will herald a new way of life for us all, ushering in a second digital revolution.

Somewhat hidden from public view, the IoT has a more sinister side. Everything we do, anywhere we go, how we get there, what we buy or consider buying, anyone we talk to or text, and even what we think about, would generate a valuable data point to be collected, analysed, aggregated and served back to us, via targeted marketing, surveillance and/or law enforcement.

The IoT includes the standard things most people have already heard about: wireless Internet-connected coffee-makers, toothbrushes, refrigerators, toasters and the like. But there are many lesser-known IoT phenomena, such as:

- 'Smart' diapers that alert you when your baby needs a diaper change: http://tcrn.ch/2HOMbjd.

- 'Fitbits' for babies to "allay parents' fears": http://bit.ly/2GOVIoZ.

- WiFi connected ingestible pills: http://to.pbs.org/2orZfmf.

- Smart pacifiers: https://www.youtube.com/watch?v=bjcVx0iD3IA.

- Robots and artificial intelligence (AI) that use and generate our personal data.

- Surveillance cameras and sensors that increasingly pepper our cities, keeping tabs on us all to 'better serve us'.

- Augmented humans, whereby technology 'enhances' human capabilities: http://bit.ly/29CITgZ.

- Micro-chipped humans: http://bit.ly/1SD3nFK.

A particularly disturbing IoT invention involves 'drones' made by outfitting a dragonfly with a tiny backpack that is then connected to the insect's brain. Humans wirelessly control the flight of the dragonfly in much the same way that humans control conventional drones (See http://bit.ly/2ov82nu).

As distasteful as these technologies are, they come with a slew of other problems.

1. With the roll-out of 5G and the IoT, our **health** will inevitably suffer due to the massive amounts of radiation being added to our already saturated environment. With 5G cells beaming radiation into our homes and communities, and all machines, appliances, devices, robots, sensors, driverless cars etc communicating 24/7, health impacts will likely reach epidemic proportions.

2. Our **privacy** is being violated by the non-consensual collection and use of our personal data.

3. Experts predict the IoT will result in **cyber attacks** far more extensive, devastating and potentially life-threatening than anything we've experienced to date.

4. **Wildlife**, bees and other pollinators are struggling to withstand the many toxic stressors—including radiation—that we have added to the environment; 5G and the IoT will likely make the situation even more dire.

5. Discarded and inappropriately recycled IoT 'things' and devices will continue to pollute the air, water and ground of remote villages in Africa and the Far East, causing serious health effects, and sometimes death, to workers who earn a dismal day's pay dismantling our toxic **e-waste**.

6. The huge e-footprint from **energy** needed to produce and run all these wireless IoT products, gadgets and platforms, will likely exceed the hoped-for and hyped-about energy-saving technologies promoted by advocates of IoT.

7. With suicide rates, depression, anxiety, autism, ADHD and loneliness now reaching epidemic proportions due to radiation exposure and screen-time addiction, adding robots and IoT 'things' to our lives may have irreversible effects on our children's **brains and humanity**.

8. In the last 20 years, **conflict minerals** used in our technology have contributed to the death of 5–6 million men, women and children from the Democratic Republic of Congo alone. What can we expect when all 'things' and appliances join the ranks of digital tech and require yet more of these rare earth minerals?

9. And what about all the ***ethical questions*** that arise from the IoT? Consider the absurdity of a new human rights law to "remain natural, i.e., 'merely' biological and organic".[50]

For eons, our inherent dependence on earth's bounty has deeply entwined us with Mother Earth. We are still reliant on the Earth for our sustenance, but many of us, hypnotized by technology, have become putty in industry's greedy hands. Telecom is now enticing and inviting us to sever the last roots that tenuously connect us to our precious earth. Playing to our weaknesses, tech companies have created a world where mainstream living means spending much of our day tethered to a digital device, with our heads in the Cloud. Tech companies, along with Google, Facebook, Amazon et al, promise us convenience, bounty, connection and even love, via e-umbilical cords that connect us all with the Cloud, while severing us from the earth.

What is progress?

True progress for our planet is not about having faster, smarter and endlessly new gadgets, but having kinder, more abiding, deeper and more fulfilling human interactions.

Testifying in opposition to the smart meter program in California, my late sister, Marti Kheel once said, "When standing at the edge of a cliff, progress is taking a few steps back." I cherish the simplicity and wisdom of her words, and would like to add to her thought: When standing at the edge of a cliff, progress is taking a few steps back, reassessing, and then forging a wiser path forward.

* Kate Kheel is a researcher, activist and creator of www.whatis5g.info.

The ultimate test of our co-creative prowess

The prospect of being irradiated from space, with no escape, is scary indeed. When we consider that 5G has the potential to wipe out many species on Earth, including humans, it's normal to be concerned—as we should be. But getting caught up in fear and anxiety only weakens us physically, while disempowering us on every level. It puts us back in our heads, worried and outraged that such things can be done to us.

While it is important to be informed so we can take whatever measures we need to take, we must remember that every crisis is a push to empowerment. Problems are not just a set of circumstances that present a threat. They are a direct reflection of what is missing in us and in our lives, clearly showing us what we must embody in order to restore sanity and balance.

We must remember that we are far more powerful than we have been led to believe, and that giving in to fear or hopelessness ensures that the other side will win.

This may be the digital age but, more importantly, it is *the age of self-reliance*. It is crucial that we reconnect with our hearts and that we engage our creative, spiritual faculties to cultivate a positive outcome.

Don't feed the scenario you fear; feed the reality you wish for.

Remember, too, that there is SAFETY in numbers. With so many of us affected by electromagnetic radiation, we can make a huge difference if we focus on what we want, rather than on what we're afraid is going to happen. Choosing to rise above the fear and to engage our higher faculties (while making our voices heard and taking assertive action) will prove to be pivotal for our world. This is not just a possibility; it is what we are being challenged to do.

Given the speed of technological advances, the colossal sums of money involved, and the quest for power that drives inhumane projects such as the roll-out of 5G, it's unlikely that words and action alone will stop it. Rising above the usual physical, conventional means of creating change, and tapping into the universal intelligence that is available to us all, may be the only thing that will turn this around in time.

When we understand the deeper dynamics of life, our spiritual essence, and what it means to be fully human, we can heal our bodies and emotional selves, while elevating our consciousness, engaging our hearts and activating our spiritual faculties to create the reality we seek.

23 Going viral

When I wrote *No Safe Place*, I had no idea it would go viral and reach so many people all over the world. Before we left Vancouver, I looked up the BC-based Citizens for Safe Technology website and found a contact in Qualicum Beach, where we would be living. This was how I connected with Marcus—our first new friend on the island and the first person I contacted about activism and advocacy relating to electromagnetic radiation. I had resisted networking as I didn't want to join a club of people suffering from EHS and then swap stories about how awful things were. I felt that would take me further down the path of being a victim, which I didn't want to be. But I needed to network if I wanted to get the word out there and have any impact at all. Plus, of course, these networks had invaluable information, support and resources that I could use to help myself and others.

Marcus had lots of great connections and he put me in touch with other activists and educators, many of whom had huge mailing lists and were in regular contact with scientists and researchers working on EMR, as well as people with EHS. He was also an excellent source of information, having spent many years working with his electro-sensitive wife Benita to create a low-EMF home environment. Sadly, for us, they were no longer in Qualicum Beach, as Benita had been unable to handle the high levels of EMFs in their neighbourhood. They'd moved three hours north, to a small town called Gold River, which had no cell towers and no overhead power lines.

It's political and economic suicide to progressively harm those who make the economy work.

But connecting with Marcus really got things rolling. All of a sudden, thanks to the many online connections I made through him, I was being bombarded with e-mails offering positive feedback and thanks for having written *No Safe Place*. People seemed to like the hard-hitting, confrontational approach versus the deferential tone that characterized so many documents and letters seeking government action. It was gratifying to think that my document had inspired others to be more outspoken and to take a stronger stand in fighting for their rights. I could see that the polite approach didn't work and that the authorities were no longer being accountable to those they were elected to serve (if they ever had been). I had no illusions about my approach working, either, but I needed to write something powerful and challenging, to reclaim my sense of dignity and self-respect.

Even though I didn't get a response from the Mayor of Vancouver or the Prime Minister of Canada, I did connect with many others who greatly increased my awareness of the scope and gravity of the situation, while also helping others to understand what was happening. I had no idea there were so many of us being affected and it was scary to realize that the authorities really didn't care that people were being seriously harmed. To me, it made no sense for a government to harm its own people and, ultimately, itself. It's political and economic suicide to progressively harm those who make the economy work. Human resources are a country's most precious commodity, so how can this approach possibly work in any government's favour? And how does this type of government differ from a dictatorship? Since the telecommunications industry and the government know about the scientifically proven dangers, how do they plan to protect themselves and their families from all the radiation, let alone the people they are supposed to be serving? While I had obviously been very naïve about politics, in the past, I now felt that politicians were being insanely irresponsible and willfully blind in their massive microwaving of the planet. I could also see that we had almost no control over the things that mattered most in life, and it was only a matter of time before the physical effects of all this radiation became too costly and too dramatic for even our delusional governments to ignore.

After writing *No Safe Place*, I couldn't seem to stem the flow. All the things I had failed to say in the past came tumbling out. I wrote to our electricity company, BC Hydro, calling them on their abusive treatment of their customers, some of whom have had their property intentionally damaged and most of whom had been lied to, had wireless electricity meters forced upon them, and their health concerns completely ignored. They were like the Mafia, solely focused on making money and forcing people to pay for an analogue meter (if they were even allowed to do that) to protect themselves from being harmed by the same company that was billing them.

Soon, even that was not allowed, and every single BC Hydro customer was forced to have a wireless meter installed on their property, regardless of the impact on their health. Despite my strong letters to the CEO of BC Hydro, citing criminal negligence and fraudulent claims, among other things, I received no reply. I followed up with a lengthy document containing 20 technical and legal questions (in addition to the rather sardonic one, opposite) for their vast team of lawyers to address, and never received a reply to that, either. Not that I expected to, but I wanted all these things to be on the record, for future reference.

If you were standing with your back to an open fire and your bum got hot, would you launch an enquiry to determine cause and effect? Or would you claim that there was no proof that the fire caused heating of the bum and that it could have been caused by the light bulbs in the room, by underground geothermal activity, or maybe even by internal combustion following consumption of a very hot Vindaloo curry?

Writing those documents felt toxic, however, as if I had somehow demeaned myself by declaring the harm they were knowingly causing, while they continued to operate with impunity and a complete lack of humanity, integrity and compassion. They had all the power and they knew it. Unless we wanted to live without electricity, and in the absence of government controls, we were at their mercy.

Having heard so much via the various EMR networks about Health Canada's claims of safety, regarding electromagnetic radiation, I had to explore this also. In my research, I realized that they were doing absolutely nothing to protect us and were, in fact, siding with the telecoms industry, just like every other branch of government. After much consultation with biologists, researchers and doctors specializing in radiofrequency radiation and EHS, I produced a document that challenged all the inaccuracies and misleading claims of Health Canada's Safety Code 6—the code that's supposed to establish safety guidelines for electromagnetic radiation for humans. The main title—*Heads in the Sand, Pies in the Sky*[51]—seemed appropriate, given their denial of the proven dangers and their failure to acknowledge what has been known about microwave radiation since the 1930s.

Not surprisingly, I received no reply from Health Canada, although they sent out a form response, months later, to everyone who had contacted them about this issue. It contained the same meaningless and inaccurate claims that we had all contested, and it only served to increase people's anger and frustration. Most shocking of all was the claim by Canada's Health Minister, Dr Jane Philpott, that even a small child using a cell phone all day long would not suffer any harm whatsoever from the radiation being emitted. Criminal negligence, reckless endangerment, crimes against humanity: they were guilty of all this and more, yet nothing was being done.

After sharing this document with the various EMR/EHS networks, I received many more wonderful e-mails from all over the world. This was gratifying, not because of the positive feedback I received, but because I was helping to raise awareness about what was going on. One of these e-mails was from a woman in Cape Town, South Africa—Denise Rowland—who asked me if I would write a letter to the mayor of Cape Town about the many cell towers being installed in residential areas and even in children's playgrounds. The poorer communities were especially affected as they had neither the education nor the resources to protect themselves or move elsewhere.

Denise sent me photos showing the cell towers located mere metres from homes and schools, and right in the middle of playgrounds, exposing small children and residents to high levels of microwave radiation around the clock. I felt compelled to help and began working on a letter addressed to the mayor and relevant city councillors. As things progressed, however, and Denise sent me more and more information, the letter turned into a 20-page document, which I called *Challenging the Towers that Be*.[52] I discovered that her older brother, William Rowland, was quite famous in South Africa, having played a pivotal role in the disability rights movement, back in the 1980s. William lost his sight at the age of four, in a shooting incident, and he became a powerful force within the disabilities movement, as well as a published author and a tireless activist. He helped to promote the concept '*nothing about us without us*', and wrote a book with that title. This was a slogan I remembered from my days as the editor for UNAIDS in Geneva, back in 2001, in the context of HIV/AIDS. I realized that the concept was equally applicable to those with electro-sensitivity—and maybe even more so. Nobody in government was consulting us about this condition. It was being ignored, dismissed and invalidated. As far as the authorities were concerned, microwave sickness/electro-sensitivity did not exist—officially, at least. To acknowledge its existence would lead to a massive public outcry and countless lawsuits. I believe that this will happen, but it may be some time before it does.

Nothing about us without us: a concept equally applicable to those with electro-sensitivity

Denise herself turned out to be a fascinating character. A former dancer, performer and showgirl, she had a rich repertoire of fascinating stories, having met and worked with many famous, colourful personalities throughout her 30-year career. The fact that Denise was beautiful, as well as a talented dancer, earned her many interesting roles.

In our daily e-mail exchanges about the EMR situation in South Africa, she recounted so many of her outrageous adventures that I told her she had to write a book. Her messages to me were deeply personal and moving, and I think they provided a safe outlet for her—a way to share details of incidents that she'd felt unable to share with others in the world of showbiz, where gossip and scandal were common currency. We were developing a close and special friendship, sharing confidences as we worked on the document together and I learned more about life in South Africa.

When I finally completed the document and Lewis had given it his usual professional finish, Denise seemed to be galvanized into action. As soon as I e-mailed the document to the mayor and councillors in Cape Town, she sent it out to everyone she knew, including those in the poorer communities being affected by the radiation. They were profoundly grateful that someone, at last, was helping them, and word began to spread. She was involved with the local EMR network (http://www.emfsa.co.za/), where she already had some good contacts, and followed up with letters to the mayor and the individual councillors. She reached out to researchers and specialist EHS doctors, deepening her knowledge and gathering data about the alarming rise in autism and cancer in certain communities.

"The statistics for attention deficit disorder (ADD) and attention deficit hyperactivity disorder (ADHD) are even more alarming, especially in sub-Saharan Africa," she tells me. "Many children are going undiagnosed or being medicated to remain in mainstream schooling. Ritalin remains the drug of choice here, even in private schools."[53]

She learned about local bylaws and who was responsible for what. In just a few months, she became an expert on electromagnetic radiation and was writing powerfully articulated letters to the authorities, exposing their corruption and hounding them with the science on EMR. I had absolutely no doubt that she would ultimately shame them into action.

Through Denise, I connected with her brother, Dr William Rowland, who was impressed by the document I'd written and wanted to help, if he could. We had several chats on the phone and it was clear to me that William was a profoundly decent, caring, wise man who was committed to helping others and to creating positive change. The honorary CEO of a multi-billion-dollar company, a board member for countless organizations, a sought-after speaker, and a seemingly tireless activist, he was still writing about disability issues, travelling widely and maintaining his many contacts all over the globe.

WHO's EMF Project is clearly slanted in favour of the very industry that is causing us so much harm. This was the head of the snake that needed to be chopped off.

Once I finished the document for Denise, I began working on one for the World Health Organization (WHO). This, I decided, was where we most needed to make an impact. It was WHO that led the rest of the world to believe that non-ionizing radiation was safe—despite the fact that their former director-general, Dr Gro Harlem Brundtland, had resigned in 2003 because the radiation from cell phones was making her ill. At the time, I was working as the editor for UNAIDS (although my contract was with WHO), right next door to the WHO building, and I was almost certainly being affected by the radiation then, without realizing it. Yet WHO glossed over Brundtland's departure and health issues, acting as if cell phone radiation were a non-issue, and setting the scene for the global denial that enabled the wireless telecommunications industry to flourish. Governments take their cues from WHO, using these claims to justify their inaction, even though they know the facts—and even though the wireless industry itself declares the dangers in the small print that accompanies its products.

Once again, it began as a letter. Three months later, I was still writing and it had morphed into a 60-page document,[54] divided into sections that documented the four key aspects of WHO's failure to protect global health. Industry infiltration; intentional ignorance; denial of the science; and disregard for humanity: they'd got it pretty much covered. (I also included personal stories from those affected by electromagnetic radiation, and a section listing what needed to be done to address all these issues and the microwave sickness/electro-sensitivity epidemic itself.) Despite the rules about avoiding conflicts of interest and not receiving funding from outside sources, WHO had been receiving laundered money from the wireless telecoms industry for decades, starting with Michael Repacholi, who was the first head of WHO's International EMF Project. Repacholi helped draft Health Canada's first Safety Code 6 and is a former chairman of the dubious but influential ICNIRP (International Commission on Non-Ionizing Radiation Protection). The current head of WHO's EMF Project, Emilie van Deventer, is an electrical engineer who has done research for the mobile phone industry. Both she and Repacholi are staunch believers in the flawed premise that only heating from EMR can cause harm. The entire program is clearly slanted in favour of the very industry that is causing us so much harm. This was the head of the snake that needed to be chopped off. I was determined to give it my best shot, even if I only succeeded in making the world aware of the truth about WHO, with regard to this crucial issue.

> "[T]he weight of evidence is that [...] radio-frequency radiation is a human carcinogen."
>
> —Dr Anthony Miller, MD[55]

As I was working on this document, I launched a 'Vote of no confidence in WHO and its EMF project',[56] which Lewis added to my website so that people could insert their name, location and occupation. By the time the document was ready to be submitted to WHO at the end of January 2017, we had almost 2,000 names on the list. This was more than any other petition to WHO or about EMR had so far achieved. (By December 2017, we had over 3,000 votes.) Many of these same people had signed up for my new mailing list. All of a sudden, I had more than 1,000 people on my list, eager for more information about what could be done.

When I had submitted couriered hard copies and electronic versions of the document to WHO, addressed to the then Director-General Dr Margaret Chan, copied to António Guterres (the new Secretary-General of the UN, based in New York) and Emilie van Deventer (the head of the EMF Project), I then e-mailed it to other relevant UN bodies, journalists around the world and all the EMR/EHS networks I'd connected with. It went viral even faster than *No Safe Place* and the response was overwhelming. Yet I was so exhausted from the effort of producing the document that I had very little energy to deal with all the messages—requests for interviews, comments and feedback, appeals for help and advice, more personal stories of loss and hardship caused by EMFs, and suggestions about what I should do next.

One of the many valued connections that resulted from this (again, via Denise) was with a journalist in Swaziland. Karl Muller was like a walking encyclopedia—an endless source of fascinating information about everything from life in Swaziland and its amazingly complex politics around HIV/AIDS, to biodynamic farming, electromagnetic radiation and its impact on young people, his plans for a radio-frequency-free zone and retreat centre, his work as a teacher who witnessed the huge rise in suicides among young black students after cell phone towers were installed, and his experiences as a musician.

Karl is also a powerful writer and, like me, an editor who works on various assignments, alongside his EMR-related activism and his multiple other projects and interests. Like Denise, he seems to be galvanized into action by the WHO document, hounding WHO for a response, citing corporate genocide and criminal negligence and tapping into his many contacts in Swaziland itself, due to the strong presence of the many international agencies and NGOs involved in HIV/AIDS.

While I feel blessed to be getting so much wonderful support and encouragement from all these amazing people, I'm disappointed that I haven't been able to follow up on my WHO document or generate a more practical outcome. Two months after sending it, I did actually get a response— something that only one other person had managed to do, apparently, regarding EMFs. Yet the response itself was meaningless—just more of the same empty claims of avoiding conflict of interest and assessing all the scientific evidence. I'm not sure what they hoped to achieve by sending this, other than inciting even more anger and frustration than they already have.

Where to go from here? How do you pressure an organization like this to take the appropriate action? It's the lack of accountability of UN agencies—as well as our lack of legal means to make them accountable—that makes this issue so profoundly frustrating.

"You've written an amazing document, unlike anything else out there," Denise tells me. "I quote your work every day. You must relax. You've done your bit, O. Let others carry on the work." I love her for saying this, and she may be right, but I can't help feeling as if I'm dropping the ball by not somehow leveraging what I've done. But it's a moot point, really, as I've run out of steam.

One good outcome is the interviews I'm asked to do. I'm particularly pleased to hear from a major EHS organization in the UK, which received funds from a private donor to do a day's worth of radio interviews, as a direct result of my WHO document. This is very gratifying news and I'm happy to do an interview, as soon as I recover some of my energy.

In the meantime, as I reflect on my options, respond to the daily deluge of e-mails and send out a newsletter asking people to follow up with WHO for some meaningful action, I notice sharp, stabbing pains in my right arm. I imagine it's because I'm doing too much mouse work (and not enough housework), and I reduce the number of hours at my desk. But the pain increases and shoots up my arm into my head, inflaming the nerves damaged by brain surgery. I'm not sure what's going on but I take out my electrosmog meter to check the microwave radiation coming off my laptop. To my dismay, it registers high levels, despite the fact that the WiFi function has been disabled …or so I thought. With Lewis's help, I discover that there is a deeper layer of WiFi functionality that must be de-activated in the laptop's device manager. When this is done, the microwave radiation levels drop down to almost nothing.

For three days, I feel utterly devastated by this. I think of the past three years that I have worked on this laptop, not realizing that I was continually exposing myself to harmful radiation, even as I produced documents designed to help reduce that same radiation in our environment. I feel utterly spent and can't seem to stop crying. All my efforts, diligence, good intentions, expensive RF shielding and careful avoidance of the radiation outside our home—it's all been cancelled out by the radiation coming at me from my own computer. (I subsequently had the WiFi chip removed from the laptop altogether.)

I take a break from all the e-mails and put the various interviews on hold. I feel defeated and used up, with nothing significant to offer all those gracious people who are impressed by my work and expect more of the same. I imagine they see me as someone capable, determined and filled with a passionate desire to nail the offenders. But that woman seems to have evaporated into thin air. I must find a way to regain my energy and motivation, and figure out how to live and thrive in this inhuman world.

24 Airlines wi-fly, on a wing and a prayer

I used to love flying. Having worked for the World Wide Fund for Nature (WWF) International in Switzerland, providing first-hand coverage of their field projects in Latin America, as well as travelling extensively for pleasure, I have lived in, worked in and/or visited 35 countries and have been fortunate to experience many fascinating cultures. Now, as of mid-2017, I'm not sure if/when I will ever fly again.

One of the most disturbing developments in the proliferation of wireless radiation is in the airline industry. Almost all airlines have WiFi on board, enabling sometimes several hundred passengers to use their wireless devices, sending multiple overlapping signals in all directions and enveloping the entire cabin in extremely high levels of microwave radiation. I don't know about you, but I'm not too keen on being stuck in a metal capsule, 35,000 feet above the ground, and being bombarded with microwaves from all sides, knowing that I'm far from being the only one affected and, given my research, that crew members (including pilots) are also reporting the effects.

Despite the fact that these electromagnetic fields are known to interfere with navigation systems, as well as potentially affecting the normal functioning of all those on board, airlines seem more concerned with keeping their customers happy and reducing the costs of entertainment technology than ensuring the health and safety for all who fly with them ...including their own personnel.

There have been many incidences of illness and medical emergencies on flights—and this may always have been true. But the number and frequency of these incidences seem to have changed since WiFi became a feature on flights. As documented in my WHO document, on 24 December 2016, a 10-year-old girl suffered cardiac arrest on an Air Canada flight and died.[57] The day before, actress Carrie Fisher had a massive cardiac episode on a London–LA flight.[58] Just a few weeks before that, 30-year-old Majella Donoghue died on a flight from Cape Town to Heathrow.[59] On 31 December, a TUI flight diverted to Shannon Airport with an ill passenger—the fourth medical emergency at the airport in just a week. The day before, a British Airways flight from Miami to London had also diverted to Shannon due to a medical emergency. On 1 January 2017, a man died on board a Kuwait Airways flight from Kuwait to New York.[60]

A leaked report about an emergency landing in Vancouver of a San Francisco–London flight on 24 October 2016 tells how all 25 crew members had to be taken to hospital. They experienced dizziness, headaches and nausea, with some exhibiting aggression, forgetfulness, confusion and the inability to think straight or converse in a normal manner.[61] Other bizarre behaviour included crew members curling up in corners on the floor, with blankets over their heads. Passengers also reported feeling unwell. All of these symptoms are consistent with exposure to microwave radiation.

Although it has been suggested that airplane fumes could have been responsible for these symptoms, it is now known that electromagnetic radiation at low intensities (that do not cause heating) damages the blood–brain barrier, allowing more toxins to enter the brain and potentially causing severe reactions and conditions. Thus, the combination of high levels of microwave WiFi radiation and toxic fumes from burning oil, hydraulic fluid or other sources can compound the adverse effects of both factors. These incidents have increased in recent years, most likely because people's blood–brain barriers have already been chronically compromised by the wireless radiation in their environment and are further compromised by the wireless radiation in the cabin.

I personally know of other incidences that remain unacknowledged by the airlines and unreported in mainstream media. I have also been told by both Air Transat and Air Canada that the levels of microwave radiation onboard their aircraft are never checked and that they have no plans to check or monitor them.

When my sister flew from Ireland to visit me on Vancouver Island, she experienced a whole week away from WiFi, cordless/cell phones and other sources of microwave radiation that she would normally experience at work and (less so) at home. Towards the end of her stay, we went shopping in Qualicum Beach, where I could always feel the WiFi in certain shops and centres. When I remarked on the radiation being particularly strong in one place, she suddenly realized that she could feel the same head-tingling sensation and cranial pressure that I normally feel—something she'd never experienced before. Then, on her Air Canada flight home to Ireland, she felt dizzy and nauseous when walking back to her seat, and she collapsed in the aisle, whacking her head against an armrest as she went down. Not surprisingly, doctors found nothing wrong and she was fine when she got home. If the incident was, in fact, due to the high levels of radiation on board (as I suspect), she is merely one of countless undocumented passengers who experience distress and malaise or worse, due to the toxic environment.

Poor air quality, high electromagnetic fields from the engines as well as from all the electrical wiring in every passenger seat (with a TV screen built into your headrest) and radiation from the airplane's radar system… that's already a significant assault on the human body without adding high levels of microwave radiation from the wireless devices used by most passengers—often for up to 10 hours, if it's a long-haul flight. An airplane is a partial Faraday cage in which the microwaves from WiFi bounce around like light off a mirror, greatly increasing the harmful exposure. It's a miracle that there aren't even more in-flight incidences, although that's bound to change as the radiation accumulates in passengers' bodies and their tolerance goes down.

Supported by WHO's denial of the dangers, coroners are unlikely to attribute such incidents to the microwave radiation on an airplane, even though scientists have warned that exposure can cause heart problems and many other serious conditions.

Even though static wicks on the wings discharge the electrical field of the aircraft to the surrounding atmosphere (enabling electricity to pass out of the aircraft if it's hit by lightning or when it builds up static electricity from flying through clouds), the EMFs in the cabin must pass through passengers' bodies, greatly increasing their body voltage and affecting their cells, blood flow, nervous systems etc. With sometimes hundreds of wireless devices in use onboard at any one time, airplanes are potential death traps for those who cannot tolerate such exposure.

It's distressing to know that I cannot fly home to Ireland to visit my parents and family—or in an emergency—without suffering severe ill-effects. Since almost all forms of public transport also have WiFi, those who are electro-sensitive are severely limited in terms of being able to travel.

Warning from the cockpit: a pilot's experience with microwave radiation on flights

In researching the science on EMR for the WHO document, I interviewed a Canadian airline pilot who had to give up her job as captain, due to being affected by the microwave radiation at work. I learned a lot from talking to her—and almost wish I hadn't discovered so much, since the facts fed my fears.

"After becoming electro-sensitive," she said, "I had to give up my career as an airline pilot because I could no longer tolerate the radar, to which I was exposed for up to 10 hours on long flights. The use of cell phones also affected me, as did the WiFi in hotels when I had stopovers. (Back then, there was no WiFi on any aircraft in Canada; now, however, there is WiFi on almost all flights, and I would not be able to return to flying.) I have personally seen a passenger cell phone unintentionally interfere with navigation equipment while in flight. There is an airworthiness directive (AD) currently in effect that requires cockpit display unit changes on B737 and 777 aircraft because WiFi is causing the screens to go blank in-flight. The AD goes on to state: *"The cause of the unsafe condition stated in the Discussion section of this AD is a known susceptibility [...] to RF transmissions inside and outside of the airplane. This susceptibility has been verified to exist in a range of RF spectrum (mobile satellite communications, cell phones, air surveillance and weather radar, and other systems), and is not limited to WiFi transmissions."* Boeing itself is patenting aircraft window-shielding to protect aircraft systems from outside microwave interference.[62],[63] If this shielding is used, airplanes would become even more of a Faraday cage, increasing the total amount of radiation within the fuselage.

"On top of this, no one is measuring the overlapping radiation from so many devices on flights, all working at full power to connect with infrastructures outside the metal fuselage of the aircraft. Nobody even knows what the cumulative radiation levels are in the cabin or whether people have put their devices in airplane mode, which many people don't bother doing. The device signals then bounce around, amplifying the exposures. All types of radiation can open up the blood–brain barrier, allowing chemicals to enter the brain that otherwise wouldn't. This, combined with pesticide use [to kill insect pest hitchhikers] and incidents of toxic air exposures that happen on aircraft all over the world, is bound to affect all who fly.

"Using this technology for passenger communication and entertainment is unsafe for the aircraft, the passengers and the crew."

Another airline pilot, now retired, had this to say:
"WiFi transmitters are being placed in the ceiling of the aircraft cabin and their locations are not being indicated or marked so passengers know whether or not their head is directly underneath one. On a long flight, the radiation from close proximity to a transmitter could exceed a safe tolerance. If a passenger has a baby on his/her lap, the danger is even more significant."

This might explain why someone walking down the aisle might be exposed to, and overwhelmed by, particularly high levels of radiation.

If you're still not convinced of the dangers, consider the feedback from Dr N. Harv Haakonson, MD, FCBOM, retired colonel and a former military pilot with the Canadian Forces, who's also a licensed commercial pilot and a Flight Surgeon Fellow of the Aerospace Medical Association:

"There is clearly enough scientific literature available to cause any experienced reader concern about the potential health and flight safety risks if this certification [changing the air regulations to allow in-flight WiFi] is done without specific study of the potential implications. [...] I do not think the potential impact on the health of passengers, and especially flight crews, has been sufficiently studied to warrant certification at this time."

25 New choices, new life

It's the middle of March and my birthday is approaching. I wonder what the next 12 months will bring and if we'll still be here, this time next year—here on the planet and here in this place. I have no vision of where we will be or how we will be living, given the plans to roll out 5G in North America and elsewhere. Our dream of having a safe place in the sun, near a nice sandy beach, is now just a faint image on the distant horizon. But it's up to me to bring it into focus and give it enough energy and positive intent to make it real.

The universe must be listening as I ponder this thought, because it seems to have found a way to help us move forward. I get a call from one of my EMR contacts—a former teacher in BC who had to leave her job because the WiFi in her school was making her ill. She made me aware of the torturous situation affecting many schoolchildren all over the country. I already knew of one—12-year-old Tyler, whose grandmother has become a friend and an excellent EMR resource to me. Tyler had to stop going to school as the WiFi was making him so ill—giving him severe migraines and night terrors, as well as causing vomiting. I had heard even more tragic stories, such as the suicide of British teenager Jenny Fry, who could no longer tolerate the WiFi radiation to which she was subjected every day in school (see Chapter 38 on children, for more on this).

My friend tells me about a large off-grid property in the interior of BC, which is being set up as a safe place for electro-sensitive people to heal. The owner is looking for a couple to help manage it. Would we be interested? We could go there just for the summer and see what we think. It would be a way for me to heal and to get away from all the EMFs that appear to be keeping me stuck in a perpetual cycle of harm–recovery–harm–recovery.

This brings up all kinds of questions and doubts. On the one hand, it's a huge gift—an opportunity to get away from all the environmental toxins and to experience life outside the electrical grid. I'm learning more about the effects of the smart grid, the dirty electricity that results, and how the voltage goes up or down, depending on what our neighbours are doing. If someone across the road is using a power saw, this can cause an increase in the electrical field and the amount of dirty electricity running through our house. Even

112

though we have removed all appliances with transformers (except for our laptops), all CFL bulbs (which emit radiation as well as dirty electricity), and anything that creates an increase on a particular electrical circuit, we're still at the mercy of what's happening within the grid and will never be fully in control of our own environment. Plus, we're told that a lot of radio-frequency radiation can also travel through the electrical wiring, even if we've eliminated all the RF emissions from our own appliances.

On the other hand, we're in a relatively safe spot (for now) and we're really only just settling in, after just 9 months. But how long will things remain this way? Already, there's talk of a new cell tower going up in our neighbourhood (and it eventually goes ahead, just before we leave). There was no public consultation and I've run out of steam for fighting this kind of thing. When I read in the local newspaper that people are saying they have a right to better cell phone coverage and that blocking the installation of new towers may even be illegal, I see that we're fighting a losing battle ...for now. This can't continue, though, and it's only a matter of time before we reach that tipping point when it all comes crashing down. In the meantime, I must do what's best for my health, even if it feels as if I'm running to the hills and being forced into a defensive position rather than making a conscious, positive choice.

But we can make this a proactive, positive choice, I tell myself. We get in touch with the owner of the off-grid property, to find out more about this potential move. She is warm and helpful, and she's had a lot of experience in dealing with EMFs and in helping others. She tells us about the property and explains the many benefits of living in a pristine environment. A writer herself, she tells me she feels intensely creative and does her best writing when she goes there.

The property is in the wilderness of the Cariboo in BC—about a seven-hour drive inland from Vancouver (which is another three hours, by road and ferry, from where we are living). The property sits high above the Horsefly Valley, through which flows the Horsefly River—the second-largest salmon-spawning tributary in BC. Surrounded by undeveloped crown forestry land, it can only be accessed via a 3.5km dirt road used for logging.

The scenery is magnificent, the owner says, and the air is crystal-clean. The wildlife is abundant, including black and brown bears, cougars, coyotes, moose, caribou, grouse and many other birds. (There are mosquitos, too, of course—and horseflies, presumably, given the name of the place. Strangely, this bothers me more than the idea of bears, as life can be hell if you're being constantly pestered and bitten by bugs. But is this reason enough not to go? Could the buzzing of mosquitoes be worse than the zapping from all the EMFs?) The wild roses, blueberries and lily of the valley are a feast for the eyes, we are told, and the place is an oasis of untamed wilderness. How often does a person get to experience that? And what would it feel like to be away from the electrical power grid for the first time ever?

In keeping with the natural environment, the property uses solar power with a back-up generator. This means that the overall footprint is in harmony with the environment. I learned from Annette that solar power can create strong EMFs as it converts DC to AC, but the owner is aware of this issue and says she has mitigated the effects. The harmonics created by a stand-alone solar-power system are very different to those coming from within the vast electrical grid, she tells me, and the EMFs from the inverter only affect two small out-of-the-way areas of the house. There are no overhead power lines, radio broadcasting stations or cell towers to disrupt natural frequencies, and there will be no wireless devices introducing disruptive signals or microwave radiation into the environment.

The owner has had her own challenges with electro-sensitivity, which means she not only understands what people need, but also recognizes the financial and logistical challenges involved in moving to a new environment. She made the choice to adopt a healthy lifestyle after finding it impossible to continue working in the city. She says she feels physically stronger and a lot healthier since making that move and that the farm work has really been good for her body and mind.

"The value of a totally clean environment cannot be overstated in today's situation," she says, "which I know is going to become worse before it reverses to sanity." I agree with this and I know that more and more people are becoming ill, whether they know it or not. "It's almost impossible for them to recover unless they leave the wireless grid," she says—and how many of them are going to do that if they don't even realize that the radiation is affecting them?

Even grounding will not help people if they ground in an environment filled with RF and extremely-low-frequency (ELF) radiation, as they become even more of a conduit for unhealthy signals. "Grounding in a pure environment is like magic," the owner tells us, "but can be the opposite in a dirty environment." This makes sense to me and also explains why grounding mats and sheets may not be a good idea. If you're in an environment with a lot of electrical fields, those fields will go through you to get to ground. The same is true of lying on the grass in an area being bombarded with man-made EMFs—which makes me think of our current situation. Although I feel a lot better and healthier in the summer, when I can lie on the grass and go swimming in the sea, I get the feeling that I'm not being as healthily grounded as I could be

After countless e-mail exchanges, phone calls and conversations exploring the pros and cons, despite some lingering doubts, we eventually decide to make the move. Yet the prospect of packing up all our stuff again so soon feels daunting. There's also the issue of Lewis's work and the clients he must leave behind. What kind of work will he do in the wilderness and will the logistics of living in such a remote place be stressful as well as expensive? Will I be able to get back to my counselling work, once I've recovered a bit?

It's a wonderful opportunity for me to write my book and for Lewis to write his second novel and get back into his art. But will we turn into hillbillies, living off the land, scratching our mozzie bites, hefting a rifle as we walk the forest trails, skinning rabbits and deer, chopping wood, chasing the neighbours' free-ranging cattle off the property, and getting stuck in the mud on the unpaved access road when it rains? These and many other issues occupy our minds as we try to figure out how to make this move without having a nervous breakdown. Can we make it work for us in positive ways, rather than it becoming just another source of stress due to the challenges of living in such a remote place? Will the benefits outweigh the downsides?

I remember contemplating our move to Vancouver Island, which was something I didn't want to do. I loved Vancouver and considered it to be my home. I did not want to go and live in a retiree community, which was what Qualicum Beach essentially was. Yet the move here had a feeling of inevitability about it, and there was no doubt that getting away from the high levels of radiation in Vancouver was the right thing to do. This move to Horsefly has that same inevitable feeling about it, although I can't yet imagine what all the benefits will be. I really don't need any more 'formative experiences'—aka *personal growth opportunities*. I just want to find a peaceful, healthy place to live so I can get my mojo back. Is that really too much to ask?

Several electro-sensitive people have told us that spending time in the wilderness did not heal their body as they had hoped. When they went back into the microwaved world, after being out of it for a year or two, the radiation affected them just as much as before. Some felt that the absence made them even more sensitive. This makes me wonder about the wisdom of moving, but I sense that it could also be a way of feeding my fear of embracing a very different lifestyle and stepping into the unknown. (We haven't even seen the accommodation we will be renting or met the owner, since travelling there and back to check it out isn't practical for us. Even a one-way 10-hour journey is daunting as I am seriously affected by the EMFs in our car as well as by the WiFi and radar on the ferry.) But I know it makes no sense to compare myself to others, since everyone has different requirements, sensitivities and ways of healing.

I sense that Horsefly holds some other gems for us, beyond the healing I hope to get from immersing myself in nature. We may make some connections there that will take us to the next step. After all, every new choice moves us forward in some way, and how we choose to be, when we are there, will have a huge impact on our experience and what we attract.

But the prospect of renting, yet again, is unappealing to us both. We want to finally have our own place and set up our own healing, empowerment and creativity centre, rather than feeding someone else's dream and helping to pay off their mortgage. On the other hand, we can probably learn a lot about off-grid living and get a sense of what works and what doesn't. Also, we must wait for some pieces to fall into place before we can realize our own vision. For starters, we have no idea where we would go, given the current situation with EMR, and I need to regain my health and get back to work so that we are financially and physically ready to take on the challenge.

To keep our own vision alive, however, and to feed our ideal future reality, we decide to draw up a list of all the elements we want to have in our ideal place—that place we've been envisioning for so long, on the beach, in a warm, sunny climate, in a healthy, natural environment. Lewis puts it all on a small poster in his inimitable creative way—a jumble of words in all directions, with colourful drawings of hearts, shining suns, ocean waves and best-selling books with dollar signs all around them. Doing this feels good. It reminds us of what we really want and that we need to keep focusing on it until it becomes a reality. With so many restrictions, due to all the radiation, it's hard to hold on to a vision of a beautiful, safe place where we don't have to think about being harmed. Yet that is exactly what we must do.

I've decided that Horsefly will be a stepping stone to that reality. I remember the owner telling me that she had seen other electro-sensitive people regain their health after being in the wilderness for 4–6 weeks, and I know that nature can do things that no practitioner or anything else can do. Grounding, negative ions, healthy air, off-grid living, fishing on the lake, learning how to use a rifle, possible encounters of the hairy kind—all of these things must surely make a difference. And since this new lifestyle will mean changing the way we do almost everything, it will change our brains and, therefore, our reality. Given the way things are, I sense the need for us to change our minds about our world ...and to change our world with our minds.

26 Human rights and human wrongdoings

In late 2017, almost a year after filing my claim with the BC Human Rights Tribunal, and having submitted a vast amount of scientific documentation confirming the harm caused by radiation from WiFi, I'm told that my case is being dismissed. I fully expected this, given what I now know about the tribunal system. The process has been a real eye-opener, but it's also distressing to realize that this entity, which is supposed to provide a fair and accessible means for individuals (including those who are electro-sensitive) to have their rights protected and enforced, is yet another smoke screen for the wireless telecoms industry.

The tribunal claims to be independent, yet its lawyers are appointed by the government. I discovered that the lawyer who dismissed one of the first EHS cases was appointed during former Prime Minister Stephen Harper's administration—the government that gagged the scientists, shunned the media, sided with industry and sanctioned numerous illegalities in favour of the wireless telecommunications corporations, allowing them to proceed with their radiation-emitting technologies (scientifically proven to cause harm) without due process, controls, monitoring, limits or any scientific testing. Yet none of this was revoked following the election of Justin Trudeau, whose father (former Prime Minister Pierre Trudeau) brought in the Clean Air Act in 1971. Initially appearing to be following in his father's footsteps, with an interest in protecting the environment, Justin Trudeau studied environmental geography (which explores the relationship and interactions between humans and their natural environment), but he quit after one year. Supporting the wireless telecoms industry, despite the huge cost to the environment and health of Canadians, the younger Trudeau shows no signs of acknowledging the harm caused by this industry or of taking steps to mitigate it.

The tribunal's corporate lawyer spent his career successfully defending wireless telecommunications corporations for a large law firm. With such a glaring conflict of interest, he should never have been allowed to hear an EHS case.

The tribunal also claims that its lawyers do not take sides. Would you trust a lawyer who has spent his career defending the offending parties, successfully pleading their case and being paid hundreds of thousands of dollars for doing so? Do you think that such a lawyer would willingly switch sides, embrace altruism and suddenly start claiming that there *was*, in fact, irrefutable scientific evidence of the harm being caused by the same corporations that he had claimed were not causing any harm whatsoever?

It is hard to comprehend how such an obvious conflict of interest, and such an egregious and transparent denial of evidence, justice and a fair hearing, can be allowed by a human rights tribunal—or any court of law.

This biased ruling sets a precedent that could prevent other EHS claimants, with valid and worthy cases, from being accorded legal assistance and from ever getting a hearing or having their human rights enforced. All cases subsequently affected by this injustice will have repercussions for everyone, far beyond the claimants involved. We all lose when justice is denied, evidence is disallowed, science is dismissed, integrity has no place, the truth has no meaning, and our humanity is eroded.

Before filing my claim, I had contacted the tribunal several times, asking what was meant by the term *independent* (as stated on their website), given the clear government bias. I asked how they could claim to be impartial, given their lawyer's conflict of interest in the EHS case. And I asked what accommodation would be provided for those with EHS, in the event of a hearing. I never received a response to any of these questions, despite my repeated e-mail requests. After filing my claim, I submitted these same questions to the chair of the tribunal, while also referring to the conflict of interest, the obvious lack of any kind of independent status, and the chain of corruption that ensured that no EHS claimant would ever get past GO. I finally received a letter in response—but it had been copied to our landlady (against whom the claim had been filed), thereby clearly spelling out for the other side the inherent bias and weaknesses in the tribunal process, which clearly compromised my case.

**We all lose when justice is denied, evidence is disallowed,
science is dismissed, integrity has no place,
the truth has no meaning, and our humanity is eroded.**

Far from being there to protect my rights or offer any kind of assistance or helpful information, the tribunal seemed intent on deflecting any kind of enquiry, exposure or attack, while dodging responsibility and accountability for its stated mandate.

The evidence submitted by our landlady was minimal and could hardly be deemed evidence at all. It consisted of three elements: 1) a blog—an example of sensationalist 'journalism', written by someone who seems to enjoy ranting about all kinds of issues, while revealing his ignorance and lack of scientific credibility; 2) a few paragraphs from the WHO website—woefully inaccurate and outdated, from 11 years ago (WHO has vastly revised its position since then, declaring microwave radiation to be a Class 2B carcinogen in 2011); and 3) four paragraphs from Health Canada's site—again, inaccurate, outdated and entirely unsubstantiated by any scientific documentation. Health Canada's position has recently been so soundly eroded and exposed for its unscientific, biased and incomplete approach to the dangers of non-ionizing microwave radiation that it would be hard to over-state its incompetence and its failure to protect our health. Health Canada itself has admitted omitting crucial scientific studies from its assessments of harm.

Clearly, the tribunal lawyers were as uninformed and as unaware of the scientific facts as our landlady—or they were pretending to be. If anyone were to read even one-tenth of the solid science, they'd have to give up their day job.

Positive precedents—and a taste of things to come?

In 2015, the Ontario Human Rights Tribunal, which recognizes that EHS is a disability and that those with environmental sensitivities, including EHS, must be accommodated, facilitated an award in *Thompson vs PUC Distribution Inc (HRTO 407)*.

Under the auspices of the Canadian Human Rights Act, it is now evident that Health Canada may be found guilty of the following charges: Prohibited Grounds of Discrimination of Disability; Alleged Practices of Services—Discriminatory Policy or Practice (Safety Code 6); and Services—Adverse Differential Treatment (not having a policy to protect Canadians against non-thermal RF-EMRs).

Human rights are primarily a humanitarian issue—not a political, commercial or legal one. But because our governments are now primarily led by industry, the respect/enforcement of our human rights is no longer a priority. Fighting for our rights has thus *become* a political issue. Contributing millions of dollars in licensing fees to our government annually, the massive wireless telecoms industry is the main reason that the public has not been informed of the dangers of wireless microwave radiation from WiFi, cell phones etc, and why people such as our former landlady are unaware of the proven dangers.

To claim that there is no evidence of EHS being a physical disability is to deny the scientific facts. And saying that electro-sensitive individuals have a psychiatric condition when they have a very real, medically proven physical one, constitutes a further violation of their rights and further discrimination.

French professor of oncology, Dr Dominique Belpomme (see Chapter 16 for more details), knows from his many years of clinical experience that evidence of this very real physical condition exists and is plentiful. He has 450 patients with electro-sensitivity and sees "20 new patients a week, including children who have headaches, impaired memory, concentration or language issues. We have the largest European cohort of electrosensitive patients. This is a major public health concern."[64]

Moreover, EHS is recognized by the United Nations and by the Canadian Human Rights Commission as an environmental sensitivity. This means it's *due to the environment*—not a mental health issue. Even if the existence of EHS had not already been medically demonstrated worldwide, the many millions of people being affected constitute more than enough proof of harm.

EHS has also been determined to be an environmental disability in other countries. In the 1960s, the Soviets recognized the syndrome of microwave sickness, documenting symptoms such as depression, sleep disturbances, headache, fatigue, memory problems, thyroid malfunction, skin allergies etc—the very same symptoms experienced by those with EHS today.

Supreme Court rules in favour of man harmed by WiFi radiation

In November 2016, the harm caused by WiFi radiation was legally recognized by a Spanish court, which ruled in favour of an Ericcson telecoms engineer made ill by WiFi at work.[65] **The Supreme Court granted him compensation for incapacity and recognized the link to radiation at work and** that the disability was solely due to ill-health from WiFi and other wireless radiation. Symptoms included headaches, tinnitus, **insomnia, memory problems, difficulty thinking clearly,** severe **depression** and **anxiety**—all confirmed by doctors in Guadalajara Hospital as being due to *"exposure to electromagnetic fields [...]."*[66]

In presenting my case, I did not need to obtain medical proof of EHS, as per the Canadian Human Rights Commission's report, which presents a legal perspective for all of Canada.[67] Nor did I need to prove that I had EHS. Legally speaking, I merely needed to identify the triggers, which I did.

There is ample evidence of the correlation between EHS and EMR, however, and the biological harm caused by exposure to microwave radiation can be seen in real time via live-blood-cell analysis.[68] Anyone denying the science is either uninformed or has some other agenda.

Since the tribunal has, as of late 2017, ensured that no other EHS cases stand a chance of winning, due to the precedent set by its industry-biased lawyer, claimants are unlikely to get legal assistance and the whole thing has been nicely stitched up.

Adding insult to injury, every rejected EHS case (including mine) is being used to further discourage any prospective individuals from filing a claim. Even pre-existing settlements are being undermined by these negative rulings, as I know from my personal connections with other claimants.

The tribunal seems to be dedicated to protecting the wireless telecoms industry at all costs, with no regard for the harm, sickness or human rights of those being undeniably affected by that industry.

It is a sad day for democracy when a country such as Canada, known internationally for its humanitarian and peace-loving stance, intentionally fails to enforce or protect the human rights of its own citizens. Despite providing refuge to thousands of Syrian refugees in 2016, it has failed to protect the vast and growing population of electro-sensitive Canadians who have become environmental refugees—fugitives in their own country who are being harmed, ignored and marginalized by their own government.

27 Invisible radiation, invisible refugees

Since 2006, I've done a variety of editing contracts for various United Nations (UN) agencies, as well as the International Organization for Migration (IOM), which has UN status. In the process, I've learned a great deal about migrants around the world and how the phenomenon of migration affects both the sending and receiving countries. Ironically, while living in Horsefly, I edited an IOM report on mobile connectivity and how vital it is for those on the move to have a cell phone and adequate coverage. For migrants and refugees all over the world, their cell phone is their lifeline—even more important than food or shelter. It's how they stay safe, how they send money home, how they find out about human trafficking networks, and how they communicate with others when they're on the move. While I usually see my editing work as a separate part of my life, unrelated to my empowerment/counselling work or my writings on EMFs, now everything seems to be coming together. Like everything else, of course, it's all connected.

As a veteran globetrotter who has worked and lived in many countries around the world, I'm already a migrant. Due to the impact of EMFs, however, I'm now also an environmental refugee, seeking refuge from the pervasive man-made radiation in our environment. I've joined the ranks of that rapidly growing sector of the population that goes undocumented, unaddressed, unseen and unheard. These are the migrants whose rights are violated and who are ignored by governments everywhere—*the migrants that nobody wants.*

A great deal has been done—by IOM, the United Nations High Commissioner for Refugees (UNHCR) and other UN agencies—to address and protect the human rights of migrants all over the world and in every conceivable situation. Those who have had to leave their homes due to natural disasters, those who have been illegally trafficked and/or abused by their handlers, and those who are discriminated against because of their race, culture, class or beliefs—all of these migrants receive consideration, protection and sometimes even legal assistance in having their rights protected. They are also increasingly given a voice, with some being invited to participate in municipal planning meetings to discuss their needs, and others being invited to share their stories in blogs or UN publications.

Yet nothing, so far, has been done for the countless environmental refugees affected by EMFs, most of whom have become fugitives in their own country, being harmed by the same governments that offer protection, financial assistance, jobs and support to foreign migrants seeking refuge from oppression, natural disasters or poverty. Most UN agencies appear to be following WHO's lead, refusing to acknowledge the existence or plight of this rapidly growing sector of the population affected by man-made electromagnetic radiation.

I decide that this will be my last assignment for IOM and I contemplate writing to the executive director to inform her about this neglected population. As is so often the case when the wireless telecoms industry is involved, many UN agencies have a vested interest in denying the dangers posed by this technology. IOM, for example, has developed an app for migrants, and its report on mobile connectivity clearly promotes the benefits of wireless technology, while completely ignoring the harmful effects. While I anticipate more of the same kind of stonewalling I've experienced with WHO and government agencies, if I decide to contact them about this, I'm also aware that I'm projecting a negative outcome onto the situation. Do I really want to compile another report about the dangers, the denial, and the human rights violations? If so, what could I do differently to promote a more favourable outcome? How could I break my own pattern of contesting injustices done to me and feeling frustrated by the non-response and inaction of those responsible?

Compiling yet another report on the dangers feels like going backwards. It also puts me back in the role of a victim, fighting for my right to exist, to live in safety and to be respected. The fight itself demonstrates that I've been prevented from doing/having all these things. Yet what kind of person would be denied these rights? What kind of person is disempowered by others? It might seem strange to look at things this way, given the nature of the threat and the power of the wireless telecom industry, but asking these questions objectively, without any emotional charge, can lead to some interesting answers. The kind of person whose rights are violated or who is disempowered by others is, in theory, someone who is weak and unable to exert a powerful enough impact to retain control over their own life and environment.

Given the current reality, this is exactly what's happening, since those of us harmed by wireless technologies tend to withdraw, defend, react and/or protect ourselves from the assault on our bodies, lives and environments. Typically, we do not seek an alternative, empowering way of addressing the issue—usually because we feel daunted by the extent and impact of what's coming at us from our external environment. *How can we, as individuals, compete with such powerful forces? What hope do we have of being heard or heeded by the massive wireless industry, which has more resources and legal prowess than we could ever hope to have?* We're so seemingly insignificant, in fact, that the industry, service-providers and government agencies can just ignore us, knowing that we can do little to stop the juggernaut of technological advancement.

In effect, we feed each other, each side playing the role that enables the other to play theirs—as in any relationship where one party is being triggered or abused by the other. It's what I call *the dance of dysfunction*—a cycle of unconscious behaviour that can keep us stuck forever, repeatedly reacting to subconscious emotional triggers relating to our self-worth and sense of entitlement. Round and round we go, accumulating more and more evidence of injustice and using our circumstances to build a compelling case against those who mistreat us. With our focus almost exclusively on our external environment, we fail to see the power of our own deeply buried beliefs about ourselves, which have more impact on our lives than anything else on Earth.

Those highly charged beliefs don't just affect us inside, reinforcing existing neural networks and causing stress, depression and conflict; with their own inherent magnetism, they radiate out into our world, attracting the people and situations that will trigger our deeply buried emotions so that, ideally, with enough awareness, we can heal them. So focused are we on what's being done to us, however, that we often fail to understand the nature of our dysfunction or what's really happening beyond our physical reality. As a result, many of us do not realize just how powerful we are or how we operate as spiritual, electromagnetic beings.

Our beliefs about ourselves have more impact on our lives than anything else on Earth.

The first step in breaking any unhealthy cycle is to stop playing our part. It takes two to keep any cycle going, but only one to break it. The dynamic is the same whether I'm in a relationship with another person or with some larger entity such as the telecom industry or government. Either way, I'm only a victim if I get caught up in the drama of the situation (giving it power over me by investing so much energy in fighting it, thereby confirming my position of weakness) or if I allow myself to be diminished or disempowered by the other party. As with most aggressors, whether they're politicians or industry moguls, their power comes from tapping into the insecurities, needs or addictions of their subjects, sure in the knowledge that most people are too disempowered, too intimidated by authority, and/or too addicted to their dysfunctional lifestyles to take any meaningful action against them.

Breaking free of our own dysfunction and conditioning is probably the most difficult thing we could ever do, if we choose to do it at all. And our pre-programmed minds will be our greatest resistors and saboteurs—even more tenacious and harmful than our oppressors. Yet, unless we take the high road of empowering ourselves out of dysfunction to a place where we can have a meaningful positive impact on our world, we'll never get to see what we're really made of.

In breaking old cycles, we must do things differently. In terms of addressing the issue of EMFs in our environment, how can I have an impact without resorting to the conventional tactics of campaigning against the industry, writing angry letters, spreading awareness of the dangers (which also means sharing and disseminating bad news), and rejecting or withdrawing from those harming me?

I know that the answers lie within us, rather than in some clever strategy for bringing down the enemy. I've done the angry rant. I've written compelling letters and taken a stand. I've filed a human-rights complaint. I've presented irrefutable scientific evidence. None of this has had the desired effect. All it has done is magnify my sense of powerlessness (while the deeper truth is that I'm being challenged to activate a much great power within me). Although some of my documents may have helped raise awareness of the issues, my efforts have not significantly changed the situation, and I've joined the ranks of those spreading the bad news. There are many wonderful EMR activists who work tirelessly to raise awareness of the dangers, and I have benefited hugely from their input. Yet if we consistently share the details of how we're being ignored, harmed and disrespected (without changing ourselves in the ways that we want the world to change), we fuel our collective failure to have a powerful impact. We also inadvertently reinforce our own self-defeating patterns, since our lack of success (in resolving conflicts, crises or any other problem) is a direct reflection of the subconscious limitations programmed into us in our formative years.

This explains why we so readily focus on the power of external authorities (and circumstances), rather than focusing on our own greatness and godness. (No, that's not a typo; I do mean *godness*—our innate capacity to change our minds, our bodies and our environment.) If we were not subconsciously conditioned to feel powerless, unworthy or unimportant, we would realize that we are powerful creators, with all the ingenuity, imagination, magnetism and creativity required to make things happen …and if we're not creating, we're just surviving, since we can't do both at once.

Our innate capacity to create our own reality is eloquently expressed by Dr Deepak Chopra in his book, *Power, Freedom and Grace*: "As a pattern of intelligence in a vast field of intelligence, you participate in creating the world you experience. The world 'out there' may appear to be objective but, in fact, the world is subjective; it is a construct of your own interpretations."

The state of our planet is a clear indication of what's trying to emerge and evolve from within.

And those interpretations come from the conditioning that causes us to perceive ourselves and the world in a limited, purely physical way. When I work with clients to transform the negative programs that so often create havoc in their lives, I never see them as being flawed or wrong. I know that whatever dysfunction they learned along the way represents the flip side of their true essence. It tells me who they are meant to be—and yearn to be— since the patterns they learned merely point the way back to who and what they really are. They are the inhibited aspects of self that are trying to break free and be expressed.

Many of us simultaneously fear and desire greatness. The same is true of success, with a fear of failure and a fear of success often co-existing inside us for decades. Even the politicians we vote for represent our attempt to be powerful by proxy. Only by looking at the circumstances can we figure out the messages. But if we berate ourselves for the state of our planet, it's just more of the same kind of negative messages that disempowered us in the first place. The state of our planet—just like the state of any relationship—is a clear indication of what's trying to emerge and evolve from within.

I see the same dynamics in the context of dealing with EMFs, which reflect those parts of self that have been suppressed. The scenario is similar; the players are just a lot bigger …which means that we are being challenged to operate at a much higher level than before.

Everyone, it seems (including me) has boundary issues, so it's no surprise that our current situation with invasive electromagnetic radiation reflects a disregard for our personal and geographical boundaries. Yet it's no longer enough to create healthy boundaries and tell our abusers that what they're doing is unacceptable (been there, done that). And it doesn't make any difference to them if we then leave (as we would any abusive relationship) and retreat to a 'safe' place (still there, still doing that). What's required now goes far beyond asserting ourselves and speaking out against an external aggressor. While our words can be powerful, there is a great deal more power in becoming spiritually and emotionally conscious and taking ownership of our situation.

Editing words and life

Having worked with words for most of my professional life, I know how much power they have. I've helped many writers and authors to make their words as powerful as possible, for maximum impact. Now, reflecting on the *vibration* of words and the emotional charge they carry, I'm aware of needing to work with them in ways that have a positive impact on my own reality. I'm therefore choosing my words more consciously, editing out any negative ones in favour of those that uplift, and using them more wisely in my life.

When we understand that we have the capacity to influence our environment, we realize that we cannot transform our reality by only focusing on external circumstances, which are merely the symptoms of our dysfunction. Catering or reacting to our circumstances, then, makes no sense …and allowing them to determine how or where we should live just keeps us stuck in a self-perpetuating cycle of reactivity and diminishing returns.

We cannot hope to have a universal impact unless we engage the higher dimensions of the self. In dealing with the seemingly insurmountable threats posed by man-made EMFs, I must therefore go beyond my limited, distorted perceptions of myself and my world. I must embrace my circumstances as a means of building greater self-awareness and empowerment, rather than seeing them as something being done to me, for some external reason, beyond my control. If I don't make this shift, I remain a part of the problem rather than being part of the solution. Since we are all connected—and all affected by what we collectively do to our environment—I owe it to me and to you to do this.

Now I just need to figure out how.

28 Interview with the EMFing enemy

When dealing with a serious issue, it's sometimes good to introduce some humour to help us retain a healthy perspective and to remind ourselves that we have just as much power as politicians (even if it doesn't always feel that way). Given the stonewalling so many of us encounter when appealing to our governments for change, we may feel that our voices go unheard. In this fictitious conversation, I've taken the liberty of expressing some of the things we may not have been given the opportunity to express, and I've had a little chat with some of Canada's finest—I'll call them Robberson, Truedough, Philpotty et al—who appear to be skilled in accidental criminal negligence, artful dodging and intentional ignorance, aided and abetted (and no doubt *fêted*) by the trillion-dollar wireless telecommunications industry. Not a single elected Canadian official/service-provider replied to my e-mails or advisories documenting the proven dangers of electromagnetic radiation and the serious harm being caused to millions of people around the world. But I know what they're going to say, anyway, so I'll just say it for them—and then everyone can see just what stellar stuff these elected public officials are made of.

ME: *Why do you stubbornly refuse to acknowledge the unprecedented amount of scientific evidence proving the serious harm caused by electromagnetic radiation?*

THEM: *There is not enough scientific evidence to prove that any harm is caused by electromagnetic radiation.*

ME: *But there are already thousands of peer-reviewed, scientific, published papers, by renowned, highly respected scientists, biologists, doctors and researchers,[69] with 20–25 new studies being released every month.*

THEM: *There is not enough scientific evidence to prove that any harm is caused by electromagnetic radiation.*

ME: *That's just denial, pure and simple.*

THEM: *No it's not.*

ME: *That's denial of the denial.*

THEM: *No it isn't.*

ME: *That's denial of the denial of the denial.*

THEM: *This is ridiculous.*

ME: Finally, *we agree on something.*

THEM: *I don't think so.*

ME: *You keep denying the glaringly obvious, otherwise known as the truth. Have you considered denying the law of gravity to see how that works for you? It would be enormously popular with everyone over the age of 30, and fabulously lucrative, although I think you'd have some difficulty disproving the validity of this particular law of physics, given the very obvious gravitational pull on certain parts of your anatomy.*

THEM: *No comment.*

ME: *How do you prove a negative? How do you prove that microwave radiation does NOT cause harm?*

THEM: *There is not enough scientific evidence to prove that any harm is caused by electromagnetic radiation.*

ME: *You're not answering the question. How do you prove that people do* NOT *have electromagnetic hypersensitivity? There's no way for you to prove that they DON'T have the capacity to withstand being bombarded with microwave radiation.*

THEM: No comment.

[Since I'm an empowerment coach who promotes healthy human dynamics, helping others to assert themselves in positive ways, without resorting to name-calling, curses or any kind of immature reactive behaviour or verbal/physical abuse, I will not allow myself to descend to that level—for example, by using terms such as *lying, money-grabbing, thick-as-a-brick, self-serving, imbecilic, brain-dead and genome-polluting degenerate*—preferring, instead, to remain respectful and mature in all my dealings with other supposedly intelligent human beings.]

ME: *Let me ask that question another way: If you were a man who had erectile dysfunction, how would you prove it? Think about it: how would you prove to* *someone that you **couldn't** get it up? You can't. (Can't prove it, I mean. I don't know about the other bit.)*

THEM: *That's preposterous.*

ME: *You mean you're too virile? Or it's too hard to prove? Listen, it's okay. If you actually do have this problem, you could probably get fitted with a wireless willy—a remotely controlled stiffy. So it could be easily fixed. Think of the endless fun you could have.*

THEM: *This is highly disrespectful.*

ME: *This is a small taste of what those affected by EMR have to endure from people like you. Not only are they assaulted by harmful radiation that wrecks their health and their lives, but they're dismissed and ignored, ridiculed and vilified. They're told that it's all in their head, they're exaggerating and they need to get psychiatric help. How does it feel to be on the receiving end of this kind of treatment, for a change? Are you feeling loved and respected by your fellow men?*

THEM: *This is far too personal.*

ME: *Really? What could be more personal than you bombarding me with microwave radiation that penetrates my environment, my home, and every cell of my body, affecting my bodily functions, hormones, immunity and nervous system, as well as my marriage, career and bank account, not to mention my friendships, lifestyle, human rights, happiness and fulfillment?*

THEM: *We're just giving the people what they want and protecting the economy.*

ME: *Well, you're certainly not giving me what I want. And if 'the people' wanted to smoke in public places again—on airplanes, in restaurants, in schools, in hospitals—you'd let them?*

THEM: *That's different. We know that cigarette smoke is carcinogenic and can kill you.*

ME: *Just as we know that microwave radiation is classified as a 2B carcinogen, which means it could potentially kill you. For the sake of argument, though, how can we be sure about cigarettes being carcinogenic?*

THEM: *Research has shown that it is.*

ME: *Scientific studies, you mean? How many, do you think?*

THEM: *No idea. Probably thousands.*

ME: *So, even though countless scientific studies have also proven (and most people with a microwave oven already know) that microwave radiation is carcinogenic and can kill you, you think it's perfectly okay to allow radiation levels to escalate without any limits, control, due process, monitoring or proper scientific measurement, bombarding babies, children, students, teenagers, teachers, workers, nurses and everyone else on the planet?*

THEM: *There is not enough scientific evidence to prove that any harm is caused by electromagnetic radiation.*

ME: *How much would be enough? I'm all the evidence I'll ever need to know that EMR is harming me, and I don't need any scientific studies to prove it.*

THEM: *There will never be enough scientific evidence to prove that any harm is caused by electromagnetic radiation.*

ME: *Of course not, because then you'd have to acknowledge the dangers. And then you'd have to dismantle the entire trillion-dollar wireless telecommunications network, roll out a much less harmful system, compensate the millions of people harmed by microwave radiation, and then compensate the millions of others whose lives and businesses have been built upon this harmful technology. You'd have so many people suing you in court that the whole industry would implode. But you're going to have to fix this anyway, in the not-too-distant future. The facts won't disappear just because you deny their existence, and bodies won't stop having their natural reaction to radiation just because you tell people there's no danger.*

THEM: *No comment.*

ME: *Here's what I don't understand: since you know that the microwave radiation from cell towers, WiFi, cordless phones etc causes serious biological damage, how do YOU plan to escape its effects? Do you think you're immune? Do you not realize that you, along with everyone else, WILL inevitably start to react as the radiation keeps increasing? Have you reserved a spot on some secret oxygenated planet, where you can go when we all start to fry?*

THEM: *No comment.*

ME: *As for 'protecting the economy', what do you think will happen when more than 50% of the population is sick and incapacitated, drugged up to the eyeballs, claiming welfare, disability insurance and an early pension, while less than 25% is paying taxes, and there's so much autism, insomnia, ADD, infertility, dementia, neurodegenerative disease and cancer that the healthcare system has completely collapsed and the government has been brought to its knees by all the lawsuits, while bee colonies all over the planet have died off, no longer providing the essential pollinating service that ensures our food supply, but everyone can get fabulous free EMFing WiFi because it's being beamed all over the planet from outer space?*

THEM: *That's never going to happen.*

ME: *You don't think so? You know this based on your extensive scientific research? Well, in that case, I should commend you for being so committed to* giving the public what they want *want (versus what is healthy and sustainable) and for so diligently, selflessly and altruistically* protecting the economy.

And, on behalf of myself, the millions of people already being affected by EMR, the millions more currently becoming electro-sensitive, and the countless others with EMR-related symptoms that remain mis- and/or undiagnosed, I look forward to a long and lucrative courtship—of the legal, multi-million-dollar, non-amorous kind.

29 Triggers for change

Perhaps it's just exhaustion from all the writing about EMR or maybe it's the stress of organizing this move, but I've been feeling stuck and lethargic, unable to gain a solid footing or move forward with my life. Have I just become so used to being ill that I've sunk into permanent inertia, or is my condition getting worse? My brain is normally so full of ideas that I sometimes feel like a traffic cop, reining them back, diverting them to a side road, or giving them enough airtime to calm them down until I can deal with them. Yet my brain has become eerily quiet and feels almost empty, while simultaneously being full of jangling nerves clamouring for my attention.

I'm pondering this when I get an e-mail from another practitioner, telling me about a therapist who does craniosacral therapy, myofascial release and scar-tissue work. Dissolving the scar tissue caused by the brain surgery doesn't seem possible, since it's underneath the skull, but I've been trying to find some way to access it. It feels as if the scarring has been pulling my neck and head out of alignment, hindering sleep and making me feel old beyond my years, with constant aches and pains. Getting old is bad enough, but growing old 10 years too soon and feeling like a full-time high-maintenance project is not what I'd envisaged at this stage of my life.

When I reach the therapist (I'll call her Tammy) on the phone, I hear a young, perky voice and I imagine a vibrant young woman, full of energy and competence. She explains her scar-tissue work and I'm intrigued. Not only is she also electro-sensitive, but she lives just outside the village in a tiny cottage with no WiFi or cell towers to mess with my head. Finally, someone in the alternative healthcare field who gets it.

Tammy is not at all what I expected, based on her voice. As soon as I see her, I feel a disturbing twinge—like a soft punch in the gut—but I need to find help and I feel I have exhausted the conventional approaches, so I push the feeling aside and greet her warmly. She's a little sparrow of a woman with a pixie haircut and a face that's seen some hard times. She's also a lot older than I expected and I wonder if she thinks the same about me. Heck. *I'm* a lot older than I expected! I can see that she's been through a lot and later discover that she has several tumours due to acute WiFi exposure. Judging from her living environment, she seems to live a simple, earthy life. She has two small dogs that greet me excitedly at the door. I'm surprised to see them in small cages in the treatment room—which is actually her living room, with a bodywork table wedged between her couch and desk. She says she has taught the dogs how to spell and that they talk to her and sometimes have messages for her clients. I'm not sure what to make of this but I accept that it's possible, in this insane world where the impossible is happening every day. I do know that I don't want them in the treatment room with me, and I ask her to take them into another room. It's not that I don't like dogs; I just want absolute peace and stillness when I'm being worked on, with no other presence interfering.

I'm aware of feeling uncomfortable and on edge. I don't like having to ask a practitioner to do what seems to me to be an obvious thing to do—to remove your pets and any other distractions when working with a client. My head is also buzzing the way it does when I'm exposed to EMFs, but Tammy assures me that there is no WiFi, no smart meter and no cell phone radiation.

Feeling conflicted but eager to get started with the treatment, I lie down on the table. Tammy explains that she can 'see' inside the body and that her hands 'go' to various parts to work on them, without necessarily moving. I surrender to the process and focus on feeling whatever it is she does. After a few moments of resting her hands on my torso, she tells me that there is scar tissue throughout my body. It's old and very dense, she says, and would cause all kinds of problems, beyond the obvious structural or skeletal issues. I realize that I've focused so much on the damage done to my brain and nerves that I hadn't really thought about the damage done to the rest of my body. But, of course, the radiation goes everywhere, potentially affecting all body systems.

The issue of invasive EMFs in our environment is all about boundaries.

While it's good to have identified another factor that has been causing discomfort, it's distressing to realize that so much harm was being done beyond my awareness. I think of how sensitive my head has become and how I've used it as an indicator of my exposure. Yet, all this time, the rest of my body has been under assault without my knowing it, and I think of all those people who never feel the radiation at all, anywhere in their body, and I wonder if something similar is happening to them.

I feel very relieved to have found Tammy (although my relief turns out to be short-lived). Even though I can't feel what she's doing when she's working on me, I sense that things are happening. After the session, I feel woolly and light-headed, as if I've got a huge powder puff inside my skull and all the neurons have been turned to mush. I can't form whole sentences and it's all

I can do to pay Tammy and weave my way out to the car where my trusty chauffeur is waiting to drive me home.

After only three sessions, I can see proof of my progress. When I lie on my back, I see that my right foot is no longer splayed out to the side as if I'm about to turn right or do some fancy dance move. My hips have also re-aligned, with the bones now sitting almost at the same level—and, I suddenly realize, the pain I've had in my back for the past two years has gone.

But this progress comes at a price—beyond the financial cost of the sessions. It's becoming increasingly clear that Tammy has serious boundary issues and most of my sessions with her have been marred by inappropriate interruptions—her answering the phone or talking about her personal stuff during the sessions and asking if I could do a documentary on her. She even suggested moving in with us. She needs to find another home and says she could work on me for a reduce rate, if we accommodate her. I find these and other comments to be so inappropriate and disconcerting that I hardly know how to respond. I'm doing my best to focus on the work and to process things afterwards and I feel overwhelmed by her insensitivity.

As I process this information at home, I realize that I'm never able to fully relax or trust that she will provide a safe environment (sound familiar?), due to her poor boundaries. I'm trying to get as much benefit as possible from each treatment, yet I'm picking up on all her stuff and trying to process and respond to what she's saying, while recognizing that the dynamics are extremely unhealthy. I tell her about the boundary issues and that I can't work with her unless she can focus on me and not talk about her personal stuff or answer calls during the sessions. On the surface, she seems to get this, but I sense that the issues has not been resolved.

While she seems to have been severely affected by WiFi radiation, Tammy doesn't seem to understand how electrical fields can affect those who are very electro-sensitive. In her tiny living room, there is barely enough space to walk around her bodywork table. The fridge is in the room with us, her laptop is on her desk, turned on and within arm's reach, and her cell phone is on, although on airplane mode. The walls are no more than a few feet away in any direction and the electrical fields make my head buzz. Even though Tammy tells me she has unplugged her appliances, I can still feel the EMFs doing a jig in my head.

I have paid up front for several sessions, and I get a bad feeling about this now. As I lie down on the table for my treatment, I'm intensely aware of Tammy's anger. I do my best to relax and set aside any negative feelings so I can focus on the work, but my body is bristling with what I'm picking up from her. After half an hour of total silence from her, I tell her I can't continue like this.

But she refuses to talk about it, backing up in the kitchen, clutching a pillow, so I gather up my stuff and prepare to leave. She nonetheless charges me for the aborted session, even though she's caused a great deal of stress and we're only halfway through. I'm overwhelmed by my deeper awareness of all these issues coming at me at once as I gather up my things. My subconscious understands exactly what's happening (and will share the details with me later), but my head is swimming as I leave and I'm horrified by the toxic and surreal nature of this experience.

I only now realize what a toll these sessions have taken. I long for Maria's gentle, healing touch. My 'gold standard' for care, Maria is a highly skilled craniosacral and massage therapist who provides a powerful blend of compassion, deep caring, sensitivity, skill and professionalism …but she's based in Vancouver. When she worked on me, every week for over a year, shortly after I had surgery, I felt completely safe and cared for. Within minutes of her placing her hands on me, I experienced a profoundly blissful peace and felt deeply loved. There was not a hint of her stuff (although, like all of us, she has her own issues), and I know that compassion and caring are just as much a part of the healing process as the work itself—sometimes even more so. Only now do I realize that these qualities have been missing from Tammy's work. I can only imagine what happened to her to make her so defensive, and I can empathize with that. But her unresolved issues made it impossible for me to relax, feel safe or trust that she would treat me with kindness.

Yet I take responsibility for my own part in this. I remember my initial intuitive sense that working with Tammy would be problematic, and I should have heeded that awareness. I compromised myself, hoping that the benefits of her work would outweigh any downside, although the reverse has turned out to be true. For me, too, it's clearly a boundaries issue. I remind myself (yet again) not to override my intuition the next time I seek a practitioner to help me resolve any physical or emotional issues. I must trust that my body knows best and let it guide me. How many painful conditions and situations might I have avoided if I had done that, all my life?

I recognize the need to further strengthen my own boundaries and to avoid making unhealthy compromises to please others or avoid conflict. When we have strong personal boundaries, we demonstrate healthy self-worth, which automatically generates healthier relationships, business dealings and finances. Further strengthening my boundaries will also, I know, make me more resilient in our irradiated environment.

It occurs to me that the issue of the invasive EMFs in our environment is *all* about boundaries. It is the direct result of our personal, physical and geographical boundaries being violated by governments, industry, neighbours etc—all of whom expose us to microwave radiation, beyond our control and without our permission. How ironic that those boundaries should be further violated by a practitioner who claims to help people heal from radiation-related harm. Even more ironic is the fact that, when challenged, Tammy reacted in the same way as many of the EMF offenders—denying responsibility, refusing to engage, and showing no compassion for the harm being caused.

I also realize something important about the effect of EMFs on my thinking and presence of mind. When my brain is scrambled by electrical fields or other sources of electromagnetic radiation, I'm unable to process this fact or find a way to deal with it. Even though I recognize the symptoms and vow to be alert to them in the future, I still fail to process the situation appropriately when I am in that mentally scrambled state. I remember attending a Thanksgiving dinner in a friend's teepee, having been assured that there would be no EMFs in the tent and that I could relax. There was a wood-burning stove in the centre, burning fiercely, with parts of it turning red-hot. Our chairs were in a circle around the fire, just a couple of feet away from it. When I got up to walk over to the food table on the other side of the fire, I could barely keep my balance and it was all I could do to walk from one side to the other without falling onto the stove. It was only afterwards that I realized someone must have had their cell phone on and that my brain was being scrambled in the usual way. Yet, because of the scrambling effect, I was unable to process the fact that I was being affected by radiation or remove myself to a safe place.

PART 3
UNCOVERING THE DEEPER TRUTH

30 Zapped ...again

There are dead bodies everywhere. They litter the floor, the packing boxes and the furniture. The smell of singed flesh fills the air and we are all exhausted from doing battle. We survey the carnage with weary smiles and sweaty armpits. It is a good kind of carnage and we congratulate each other on a job well done. There will be more to come but, for now, we've dealt with most of the invaders and things are relatively peaceful. It's not exactly what I had envisaged for our first few hours in Horsefly.

We had arrived, dizzy with fatigue after 10 hours on the road, silently praying that all would go well. The 3.5km driveway to the property was like a moonscape, with thick clouds of fine dust billowing up all around us, major potholes and rough terrain. Our minivan could barely deal with it and it was hard to tell what colour it was when we finally pulled up beside the house (a really nice shade of turquoise, in case you're wondering). Our truck driver had got there ahead of us and was already unloading our belongings with the help of the owner and her young handyman.

But, when we went inside, the seething mass of mosquitoes that greeted us was a real shock. Even in my travels to the tropics and through the Amazonian jungle, I'd never seen anything like this. They were swarming, teeming, filling the air around us, covering the windows and attacking all exposed skin with great gusto. I could not exaggerate if I tried (and I'm quite good at exaggerating, although that's probably a monumental understatement).

Thankfully, the owner came to the rescue and prevented me from running screaming down the driveway, happy to be mauled by a bear, attacked by a cougar and put out of my misery with one fatal blow. She handed us both an electronic mosquito-swatter that looked like a tennis racket. When all the furniture was in and the doors closed, we all began madly swiping the air, killing hundreds with every swing and producing a very satisfying zapping sound. This helped defuse some of my terror at the prospect of having to live with this perpetual torment, not to mention all the pent-up anger and frustration of having had to move to this wild, inhospitable place because so many uninformed humans were zapping *us*.

But the mosquitoes turn out to be a minor, short-lived irritation in the bigger scheme of things. I've been feeling another kind of buzzing in my head since we arrived—an all-too-familiar sensation that I normally associate with EMR exposure. I couldn't even think about this the day we arrived but, the following day, I take out my electrosmog meter and my body-voltage meter and do some testing. To my dismay, I discover high levels of electrical fields throughout the unit and, not surprisingly, high body voltage. There are extensive fields coming off the Internet/phone router and they seem to permeate both units, even when the Internet cable to Unit 2 is unplugged.

This is a devastating blow and we can't even begin to process it. We've come here to get away from the man-made radiation back in the so-called civilized world and have committed to being here for at least four months, yet we're right back in the same exposure–avoidance dynamic that we left behind. In fact, it's even worse. We gave up a relatively stable situation where we had control over our living space and had managed to shield it from the neighbours' WiFi and smart meter emissions. Yet this house seems to be less EHS-friendly than what we left behind.

Dazed and in a state of shock, we sit down with the owner to discuss the situation before she heads home. It becomes clear that a big part of the problem is the dirty electricity coming from the solar panels beside the house. Solar power is known to produce significant levels of dirty electricity because of the inverters used to convert the DC solar energy into AC current.

To avoid the dirty-electricity issue, solar panels need to be connected to a battery outside or in a separate building from one's living space. Instead, here, the power comes into the house via the master bedroom, where we sleep. So, as soon as the sun comes up at 5am, I'm wide awake and feeling zapped by the strong currents going through our room to the battery in the laundry room at the front of the house, where the inverter is located. This is simply not going to work and we don't understand why this issue has not been addressed.

The satellite Internet connection also seems to be a problem. When we were part of the grid in our last place, there were significant EMFs coming from all the computer equipment and Internet router in Lewis's office, but they did not extend beyond that room. Here, the fields seem to extend throughout the whole house, even in those rooms with no Internet connection or cable running through them.

We're too exhausted to think clearly or to contemplate our options. The owner, trying to be helpful, suggests that I stay in the small cabin on the property, as it has no electrical power and provides a clean EMF environment. This seems like a good option, at first, but it quickly becomes clear that I don't have the reserves for this kind of primitive living. There is no running water, which means I must carry it over from the house, or get Lewis to do it for me.

There is no toilet—just an outhouse about 50m away. Using this is a novel experience for me and one that I find rather sphincter-clenching. I don't like to think of myself as being anally retentive but how can you *not* be when your naked bottom is perched over a 30-foot shit-pit, with mosquitoes and other blood-sucking varmints making a bee-line for your tender buttocks.

"How can anyone possibly let go, in those conditions?" I ask Lewis.

"Letting go is your only defence," he says, and we dissolve into much-needed laughter.

But living in the cabin is no fun, and it's certainly not what we signed up for. For starters, my man is still sleeping in the main house as there's not enough room for him in the cabin's double bed. And the logistics of this kind of living require a huge amount of energy and resilience. It might seem quite bucolic to get *back to nature* and to be cooking outdoors on the barbeque, but when you're being eaten alive by mosquitoes, when the gas burner keeps blowing out in the wind, when you have to walk back to the house three times to fetch something essential you forgot, and when you're so depleted that just dropping your fork on the floor is enough to make you cry, it's really not conducive to healing or relaxation.

What the heck are we doing here? How can this EHS 'sanctuary' be worse than what we left behind in the 'normal' world?

In desperation, I reach out to some of my EMF contacts—one, in particular, who has long-standing experience with off-grid living and a solid knowledge of how things work.

"Recreating everything that's wrong with the grid in the middle of nowhere is not a sanctuary," she says, after I describe the set-up here. "In addition to the dirty electricity from the solar power, the radio frequencies from the satellite Internet connection create a truly absurd, off-grid hell."

Kicking myself for not having consulted her about all this *before* we moved here, I digest her advice and suggestions about what can be done to make this a healthy, safe place to live.

For those, like us, who are renting a solar-powered property, my friend recommends the following interim measures:

a) If the system is AC (not a 12-volt system set up intentionally as DC, which is clean), then the inverter, which inverts from DC batteries and DC panels to AC wiring, needs to be shielded—or, rather, the inhabitants need shielding from it, unless it is a pure sine wave inverter. Any modified sine wave inverter is sickening.

One can create a cheap but effective Faraday cage very easily for the solar system (although you don't need shielding for the cable, the panels or the battery bank, which is DC and generates no fields). If the solar system is properly set up, the cable connecting all the components would be armoured and would present no problem either. (This is not the case here, but resolving this would require considerable investment by the owners.) As an interim solution, the solar unit should be completely enclosed within a cage made from aluminium mesh, with a wooden frame. There must be no gaps, staples or anything else penetrating the shield. Electrical tape should be used and only uncoated genuine aluminium insect screen.

b) Use a shielding canopy over the bed, with an under-bed mat, if necessary. Or shut off all the power every night. Food in the fridge will keep overnight just fine, but it's best to turn off the inverter when you go to bed.

c) A sine wave tamer should handle the rest and prevent re-radiation back to the solar array or on from the circuit box into the wiring throughout the house. (See Chapter 59—Holistic help for the body: what worked for me—for information about sine wave tamers.)

Before the owner leaves, she takes Lewis on a small tour of the woods around the property, past the beaver dam and the moose-grazing fields, although they have no sightings of anything larger than flying insects. When Lewis returns, he has so many mosquito bites on his forehead that he looks like a primitive, brooding Cro-Magnon man. He looks so distressed and fatigued that I want to bundle him up and take him to some luxury resort on a remote tropical island, away from all this madness.

Once the owner leaves, we are left to our own devices, trying to figure out how to do what we came here to do. There is another couple in the other half of the main house (further away from the radiation being emitted from the inverter and satellite dish), and we decide that we will move into that other unit when they leave at the end of the month. In the meantime, I will have to stay in the cabin, getting as much grounding on the earth during the day as I can, and taking advantage of the natural environment around us.

Sadly, this will not be the EHS haven that the owner envisaged, unless the solar-power system and Internet are re-configured so that no EMFs pollute the living space. Things are not going according to plan—for us or for her.

31 Stripped of distractions

I am proud of Lewis and profoundly grateful for him. I see him trying to be strong for me when, in fact, he is close to cracking from the strain. This makes me determined to be very strong for him and I feel ashamed at having been such a cranky wimp since I got here. I've done nothing but complain about what's not working, rather than seeking to understand the deeper truth, as I normally do. I know there is always a deeper layer of reality trying to get my attention, and that every situation holds the gems of another breakthrough. I brought myself here, after all, so there must be a good reason for it. I can see myself as being naïve and dysfunctional (which I may be), or I can see myself as being intuitively inspired and gamely striving for something unexpected on the other side of these seemingly daunting challenges.

It would be so easy for us to spiral down into despair, and we've come close a few times. It's also tempting to see this move as a monumental mistake and to have bitter regrets about having come here. But I want to see it as a stepping stone to something better. After all, I can only get to the next place from where I am, and I am here. Even if it's not our ideal place, making it *right* will help us to attract the best place. If I live in a state of being in the wrong place, I will attract more of the same. If I live in a state of always being in the perfect place, I will attract more of that. So I know I must stop resisting our current reality and surrender to it so that its benefits can become clear. I must *be here now* and be grateful for what IS here, rather than spending all my time trying to be somewhere else. This feels like a familiar theme—always being on the run, in search of something better—and perhaps it's an issue particularly for those who are electro-sensitive, as they are often forced to move in search of safety. It may also be true that we are running from some denied part of ourselves—a denial or self-rejection that weakens us or makes us vulnerable to outside attack.

Whatever the case, it's a reminder to be present—a state without fear, negative projection or anxiety. I know that peace is inside me, not out there in some magical, perfect place. I can tap into it now, here, and make it a part of my life, even though things do not seem conducive to me feeling peaceful. It's another of the many ironies I'm perceiving here—how hard we sometimes have to work and how much we struggle with ourselves and our inner demons in order to be at peace. Yet letting go should require no effort at all. It's just our conditioning and the resulting negative expectations that keep us locked in a state of angst.

I realize, too, that being fearful has far more to do with fear itself than with what we might be afraid of. The same is true of being nervous, which is really the same thing—just another degree of fear. When the nervous system is constantly agitated, whether by EMFs or something else, it can become locked into a state of nervous tension and become vulnerable to whatever might trigger it. Back on Vancouver Island, my anxiety was centred around the radiation coming at me from WiFi, cell towers etc. Here, my anxiety has expanded to include the prospect of meeting a bear with a grudge, a cougar with attitude or even one of those large black spiders that creep up on you and give you a nasty bite when you're trying to relax and watch a movie.

**It's ironic how hard we sometimes have to work
to be at peace.**

The stress created by fear and anxiety gets in the way of healing, and it's clear to me that I must find that inner peace, regardless of where I am. That, in itself, could be everything.

Being here is also causing a shift in our priorities. Given the unexpected challenges we've had here, I now feel that having a home of our own is the most important thing. We would never have considered buying a place out here, miles from the coast, in the remote countryside. But if we can find a comfortable place with enough acreage to create a healthy buffer from wireless-loving neighbours, and with a separate space for Lewis to set up an art studio, it would be a huge relief. To have control over our own environment and to be able to invest our time and efforts in a place that's ours would also make a lot more sense—particularly with the ongoing increase in property values and the fact that it may be several years before governments come to their senses and recognize the need for less harmful telecommunication technologies.

***

It feels as if the whole world has fallen away. It's an unfamiliar feeling that causes lots of probing questions and uncomfortable emotions to rumble up from within. Who am I, when all my familiar landmarks are gone and all those things that define me—work, neighbours, daily interactions and emotional triggers—are stripped away? As I exist in what feels like a vacuum,

I'm challenged not just to reinvent myself, but to decide who I am when all this 'stuff' is gone. I get to see how much of me being me is really me being a reaction to external things. If I take away all my reactions—to e-mails, to what people say, to what's happening in the world, to the 'injustices' of our situation and to how I might be feeling—what's left? And is whatever's left the authentic me?

What *is* left? I'm not even really sure. What parts are the real me? How do I define myself when I don't have other people around me to relate to? We do, in fact, still have the other couple living here on the property—for a few more weeks, at least. They are retired teachers who used to live a very comfortable life south of Vancouver, but had to give it all up when the wife became electro-sensitive. They, like so many others, have moved numerous times, trying to find a safe place to live. It's been great to have them here and their input has inspired me, in several ways, reminding me of the need to meditate and to focus on the positives.

But they will soon be moving on, to a ranch south of here where they rent a large wall tent every year. While it's been wonderful to have some company and to share our experiences and resources, I realize that it may also be a way for me to stay stuck. Before moving here, I promised myself that I wouldn't talk about the challenges of living in the microwaved world. I would leave it behind mentally as much as I had left it behind physically. Yet I haven't done that, and I see how easy it is to use others to echo my fears and frustrations. When they leave next week, I will be sorry to see them go, since we will be truly alone on this 164-acre property, in the middle of nowhere. On the other hand, I will get to hear the echo of my own thoughts, without the distraction of someone else's input. There will be no one to validate my sense of injustice or to reassure me that I'm entitled to feel this way. While there is kindness and support in this kind of sharing, I'm aware that I'm still justifying my sense of having being wronged, harmed and evicted from the life I consciously chose.

32 Exploring new dimensions

I'm tired of my story—the *I've-had-a-brain-tumour* story. I do not want to keep feeding this story of harm or to be known as a brain-tumour survivor. In fact, I don't want to be known as the *survivor* of anything. I'd like to be known for doing something extraordinary—overcoming my challenges in some creative way that will inspire others to do the same. I want to learn how to thrive in an environment that temporarily threw me into survival mode and made me question my purpose, my power and my right to exist. All of these things are, of course, designed to push me in the opposite direction—to embrace my purpose, to express my power and to claim my right to thrive.

I have always been fascinated by the plasticity of the brain and the magic that comes from being creative and tapping into universal intelligence. I've been reading the books of Dr Joe Dispenza[70]—a chiropractor who healed his own severe spinal injuries, using the power of his mind, neuroplasticity and the principles of quantum physics. As I gain a deeper understanding of the quantum field, neuroscience and the brain's plasticity, I realize that the principles are similar to what I've been teaching about the subconscious mind. But I haven't been applying these principles as fully or as mindfully as I should, in order to create the outcomes I want, and this work takes me much further along the path. It's not just about understanding the negative subconscious programs that drive unhealthy behaviour, or changing that behaviour in order to change how we think and feel, as well as what we manifest.

I must completely change my thinking and my habitual way of doing things. All repetitive thoughts and actions must change in order for my external reality to change. This could mean brushing my teeth using my non-dominant hand (not as easy as it sounds; my upper lip ended up cleaner than my teeth); choosing to say something positive about someone (including myself) I might normally criticize; catching myself if I'm about to repeat some tired old story; staying silent unless I have something meaningful to say; and doing the cha-cha on the way to the clothesline to bring in the washing. (Yes, some people do still use a clothesline.)

New neural pathways—and, consequently, new possibilities—can only be created by actively breaking old habits, doing new things and thinking/

146

behaving differently. This, in turn, primes the brain to interact more powerfully with the quantum field, generating new opportunities and realities. Neurons that fire together wire together, which means that repeated negative thoughts and/or actions solidify existing habits and tend to keep us stuck in unhealthy behaviours. Likewise, "neurons that wire apart fire apart," says Dr Norman Doidge, in his book, *The Brain's Way of Healing*, and this enables us to "undo brain connections that are not helpful."

It can be difficult for the mind to accept that this is possible, given the alarming nature of our current environmental threats, but these principles are just as valid in terms of protecting ourselves from EMFs. Feeding the story about the harm they cause makes us even more vulnerable to harm, whereas creating a new story about safety, resilience, freedom, mobility and health primes the brain for greater resilience and starts to create a new reality featuring all of those things. The story begins in the mind but it ultimately becomes a physical reality, if we understand the quantum laws and consistently apply them in our lives. This means that it's not just about changing ourselves but also our world.

Dispenza explains how repeated negative emotions, projections and fears create stress chemicals in the body, which then re-create the same negative feelings as before, keeping you stuck in a perpetual loop of emotional addiction. These chemicals create and feed neural networks that become so deeply entrenched that they start to run the body and to tell the mind what to think. This makes perfect sense to me as I've become acutely aware of the physicality of some of my feelings—particularly those relating to the dangers of EMFs, which can trigger a fight-or-flight response that throws the brain into a defensive survival mode. I've been working on this for some time, aware of the need to cultivate a sense of inner safety, even if the external threats persist. If I repeatedly tell my brain that I'm safe and resilient, it will make the necessary adjustments to ensure that this is so. In other words, it will cue my body's immune and nervous systems to more effectively protect me from external harm. It will also make the switch from a heightened state of defensive alertness, to a relaxed state of inner safety and peace.

**If I repeatedly tell my brain that I'm safe and resilient,
it will make the necessary adjustments to ensure that this is so.**

While I understand the concept, I'm not quite there yet, and it requires a supreme mental effort for me to override the usual arguments when they kick in, trying to pull me back to the familiar feelings of injustice that have coloured so many of my experiences in life. *She had no right to treat me like that. He always over-reacts to things.* Even though these claims may appear to be justified, I know it doesn't serve me to dwell on them. It's stressful and toxic and I'm ultimately only harming myself, while also keeping myself stuck in a cycle that's preventing me from healing. I know this is part of some old inherited pattern—the belief that there will be a price to pay for taking care of me or trusting someone else to help me. Now that I understand the science and biology behind it, I'm very motivated to get it out of my system. Every time the same old refrain kicks in, I interrupt it with a simple phrase that seems to instantly defuse all the angst and indignation: *Peace in the body*. Every time I say this, my body softens and relaxes, making me realize just how much those toxic thoughts have been affecting me. I keep doing it until the 'victim voice' has faded away and I've expunged the negative feelings from my body.

If we have nowhere else to go but inside ourselves, we are forced to access our higher faculties to rise above a reality that we cannot seem to change with words or activism alone.

I realize that I must also create a clear mental image of an ideal future reality and start being delightedly grateful for it, as if it already exists. Although the process sounds similar to doing positive affirmations, it's much more than that. The brain itself must change so it can start to create the new reality I desire. In embodying the appropriate elements of proactive change, positive intention, excitement and gratitude, I can access that desired potential, out there in the quantum field, where all potentials already exist. It will then materialize—becoming matter and taking physical shape in my world, as a result of me changing my mind in order to change my reality. This, I believe, is the higher calling inherent in the challenge of dealing with the impact of electromagnetic radiation. If we are being harmed and have nowhere else to go but inside ourselves, we are forced to access our higher faculties to rise above a reality that we cannot seem to change with words or activism alone.

Some people feel that healing themselves would let the offenders off the hook. *If we are no longer so affected by the radiation, then industry, governments and service-providers can just keep doing what they're doing and will never be held accountable for the harm they've caused.* True. But do we really win if we remain stuck in a state of ill-health and victimhood? And there's still the harm being caused to plants, animals and our environment, so it's about more than just us. The effects of applying quantum laws go far beyond us healing or strengthening our bodies.

Healing ourselves, while feeding a vision of a healthy environment, will ultimately *generate* that healthy environment. It will create a win–win situation. We will protect our bodies while helping to build a healthier world using the power of our minds and tapping into universal intelligence. Everyone will benefit and we will have the opportunity to demonstrate the human capacity for enlightenment and empowerment to those who are temporarily disconnected from their own personal power. Addicted to the much shallower and less fulfilling connection via their wireless devices, they cannot yet see what is missing within themselves or in our world. Nor can they see that their actions are self-destructive, since our planet will not be able to sustain us if the growing EMR assault continues. We all have the opportunity to show each other that, while reminding ourselves that we teach what we most need to learn.

33 Pondering the deeper truth

We're sitting in the cabin, swatting mosquitoes, eating barbequed elk burgers, and contemplating what it means to be here, alone in the wilderness. What defines us, now that all those things have been stripped away?

"I'm not sure I know the answer to that question," says Lewis, "although maybe I'll discover it here."

"Well, it would be good to not just be a reaction to what's happening," I say. So far, I feel that that's exactly what I've been—an emotional, dramatic reaction to what appears to be a disastrous situation. We could get great mileage out of that at dinner parties, rolling our eyes and giving dramatic accounts of *that dreadful time in Horsefly*—when we were devoured from head to toe by hordes of savage mosquitos (and only our eyeballs were spared), bitten so badly by monstrous spiders that we could hardly walk, got stranded in the woodshed in the middle of a force-10 gale, had to evacuate to the village church when a wildfire threatened to consume all our worldly possessions, couldn't reach civilization when the road got flooded under six feet of water, had to scare off a cougar on the lawnmower (I had no idea that cougars knew how to use those things), and couldn't get the bear cubs off my trampoline so I could use it. Okay, so we'd have to take a bit of dramatic licence to make it worth the telling, but I don't think that's why we're here.

"If everything we *do* is gone, as well as all the platforms for doing what we usually do, we're left with a void that must be filled in some other way," I say. "So it's an opportunity to step into that and *choose* who we want to be, isn't it?"

**We can impose our own positive spin on things
and let that define us and our world.**

I think of the principles of quantum physics that we've been reading about, and I know they apply here as much as everywhere else. *It's time to be defined by a vision of the future*, says Dispenza, *instead of the memories of the past*. That's it, in a nutshell. Regardless of what's in front of us now, we must invent a new future for ourselves, in our minds, while fuelling it with excited anticipation and gratitude for how amazing it is (out there in the quantum field). We must be greater than our environment, as Dispenza says, and greater than time, which means that we must be *ahead* of our time.

Being here is challenging us to creatively step into our gifts and really use them. It's also an opportunity to strip away who we used to be, and then come forward from a new place, building something on a cleaner foundation. I think of the wooden houses in Western Canada—houses that seem to be built in a matter of weeks—versus the solid brick or concrete houses found in Ireland and other parts of Europe. In Vancouver, we often witnessed older wooden houses being stripped down to their wooden skeletons and then covered up again with a new exterior. Yet nothing had fundamentally changed. They'd just had a cosmetic facelift.

"A new environment challenges you to look at things differently so that you have to come up with something new," Lewis says. "It also challenges you to dig deeply into yourself to find your strengths, be a bit braver and take more risks with yourself. So you're stepping outside your own box."

If you strip yourself right back to who you really are, you connect with something deeper—your soul or spirit or universal intelligence, which is what you tap into when you're really inspired and have a vision of something bigger than yourself. And, when you do that, you're opening up to a much vaster bank of resources—and it doesn't matter where you are. Those resources are always there inside and out there, in the universe.

Ironically, we tend to think of being deprived of things when we're in a remote place like this, but the opposite can, in fact, be true. By tapping into our deeper selves and the universal intelligence available to us all, we can essentially amplify our resources, whereas we limit ourselves if we just use strategies or systems that have nothing to do with who we really are. In a way, those strategies can cover up the parts of us that we only get to see when we strip away all the externalities.

We can intellectually know this stuff—the power of universal intelligence, the fact that it's there for us all to tap into and that we don't have to do all this alone—yet still not really embrace it or trust that this greater power is real and reliable. Is it just our deep conditioning—the belief that it's safer to have systems in place—that keeps us from tapping into that universal intelligence?

Many of our personal defences are the result of a subconscious rejection of self. We only worry about not being accepted if we have issues around feeling worthy, which can cause us to make unhealthy compromises in the hope of gaining acceptance, validation or approval. This means that we ourselves often impose the limits that we think are being imposed on us by others.

If we recognize what's really driving our behaviour, we can do the same thing in the other direction—impose our own positive spin on things and let that define us.

I think of our good friend Adam, who has a passion for making car-bikes, and who is now helping someone build a tiny home, and is also running a business selling bone broth—all of which came about because he just loved doing those things. He never stopped to wonder if they would fly or make money. He never cared what people thought and never worried about others judging him. He just did these things because he had a passion for them— and they are all potential money-makers. There's a sweet innocence in that way of living that I really love. I used to live that way, not so long ago, but I realize that I've become hardened in my battles with EMR and my perception of the world now being an unsafe, unfriendly place.

If we cultivate an expansive thought and allow our bodies to get used to that freedom, it can change everything.

Breaking free of old limits requires being consciously aware of what we say, think and do. It all starts with words, which have a charge behind them, and those words then create a feeling, which then creates an experience and an outcome. We must chose new words and ideas to describe or think about ourselves, if we are to change our personal reality.

If we cultivate a new, expansive thought and allow our bodies to get used to that freedom, it can change everything. So much of what we do starts in the head and then descends into the body to create visceral feelings and reactions. Yet those feelings and reactions are now running the mind and they have very little to do with who we really are. If we want to be truly different and to become something new, we have to change those fundamentals. The person we think we are may be nothing like the deeper, authentic self trying to burst out.

The gap between where I currently am and being healed and healthy can seem huge. Yet bridging that gap can be easier than we imagine. It could be as simple as consistently expressing and embracing positive new statements that describe an ideal reality.

Once again, the same can be true for EMF-related health issues. I think of some recent conversations I've had about the EMR situation, and I hear myself saying the same old things. What can I say differently that would completely break the pattern of this conversation? Obviously, I can talk about solutions and mastering the body and mind so that the EMFs no longer affect me. Yet the mind gets stuck in a rut and we often use others to keep ourselves stuck in that groove. *She won't understand what I mean if I say that. He's a scientist and he's not interested in this way of thinking.* But it all comes back to self and the clever strategies we use to continue being who we think we are.

To change this, we must become conscious of the patterns, the same old words that confirm what we already believe, and the *lippage* (which I define as unnecessary, unimportant words that really don't need to be said—flapping your lips, expressing inanities and stuff that does nothing to take you forward in your life). When I do this, I gain a deeper recognition of the superficial stuff that looks like life but really isn't life at all.

It's about daring to go beneath the surface and asking deeper questions. *What do I mean when I say that, and what does that say about me?*

Who am I if I take away the idea that I've aged horribly? Who am I if I let go of the idea that I've got to be an activist and to respond to all these wonderful people who contact me and ask me to talk about EMFs? And what is it that drives my desire for justice …and is it also a desire for revenge? Do I feel, deep down, that the world needs to pay me back for what's happened to me? How can I know where I'm truly coming from, in the midst of so much disturbing, distracting stuff coming at me from the outside?

Lewis doesn't think it's about revenge. "You have a very strong voice in this area," he says, "and I don't think it is about revenge."

"I'd *love* to get revenge on certain people …sometimes," I say. "I can't be angelic *all* the time, you know."

"But the way I see you going about it has more to do with the issue and the harm that's being caused to so many people, including you."

"I get that, and that's one layer of reality, but there's a deeper layer driving that—whatever caused me to be in this situation in the first place."

"So what's that about?"

"I'm wondering if, in this state of electro-sensitivity, there's some suppressed part of the self that creates vulnerability. Many of us develop insecurities and then believe that we can't have what we want. It's different for everyone, I know, but I get the feeling that all that EMF-driven stuff physicalizes into challenges that push us to become powerful in particular ways, beyond the issue itself."

"I think you're suppressing yourself by not allowing yourself to be powerful," Lewis says. "You got a glimpse of that by producing those documents, and then you backed off because of the way you're feeling and the projections you have about yourself. I think that's a bit of a pattern. You take it so far and suddenly people are taking notice of you and you back off. I think you'd get a lot more satisfaction if you kept going and ran with it. Let people interview you. Let your voice be heard. Then you will start being the person who has the power, rather than the person who's the victim, at the effect of all these things. Instead, you become a person who's creating an effect, and that is what power is all about."

My ego certainly likes the sound of this, but is that the deeper truth?

"You're right. There's an opportunity to leverage what I've done and to take it to the next level, and I'm not really doing that. But I also see that I can get very intense and invested in the process, going on a crusade and loudly proclaiming the injustice of it all and what needs to be done to make it right."

"But you're now talking about what can be done, which involves raising awareness of the harm, but it's not protesting it; it's informing, and then introducing and inviting solutions. It's not a victim thing; it's a clarification of things with a focus on solutions. It's about transcending that state of stuckness where so many people find themselves. You're no longer interested in a victim evidence-gathering process. You have the opportunity to create a powerful movement and a deeper understanding of this whole situation that's so much better than just whining about it."

It disturbs me to contemplate this pattern of not following through when I reach some critical point, which I do recognize. *Why are we afraid of being powerful?*

It's a pattern that can be exhausting and unfulfilling, and it doesn't serve anybody. However, I sense that there's value in stepping back from it all and writing my book, in that new vein. That doesn't mean I can't have conversations about EMR, such as with the company in Europe that's doing a documentary on those living with EHS. At the moment, though, I feel I've run dry. I don't know if it's because I got over-exposed to EMFs again without realizing it, or if this is a healthy pulling back so that we can have these conversations and come to some deeper realizations about what's really going on …and then come back out with something that's more complete.

I don't feel I can push myself to engage. I don't even want to do any of the other things I planned to do—such as doing an exposé of the EMFs on airlines or a video to Justin Trudeau. In forcing myself to do those things, I feel I'd be feeding the conflict and giving them a lot of power over me. Grappling with all these external mechanisms, such as the Human Rights Tribunal, is just a way to keep proving to myself how awful things are, that nothing works and that I appear to have no rights. Those mechanisms have proved to be useless, yes, but maybe that's the way it's meant to be, because all that's left then is me. So I want to come from a more autonomous place, to resolve that deeper conflict within myself, and to find peace, regardless of what's going on out there.

"Well, maybe you could also look at it slightly differently," Lewis says, in his usual considered, thoughtful, heartfelt way.

"I will and I do and I love you," I say, because this man has been with me every step of the way, despite the grueling challenges, all the moves, the huge cost to his career, and the curtailing of our lives on every level. He's been there when I've hit despair, questioning the point of it all, why we are here, who needs this, where's the joy in this, when will I be on a beach again and will I ever not be cranky about someone two feet away from me yakking on their cell phone? Yet these are all the negative projections that I need to let go of and replace with their opposites.

"You can see some of those interview opportunities as a platform to share these deeper insights. You don't have to keep repeating that same old stuff about how harmful EMFs are. Tell the story that *you* want to tell and use it to flex those new mental muscles so that you continue to build in the direction that you want to go."

"I like that and I know that being asked questions always brings out things I didn't even know I knew. But I must also actively engage enough in that new story that I'm inspired to have that conversation. I feel there's value in investing energy into the emerging me, until I feel energized enough to express whatever's trying to evolve." And I do feel that there's something bigger trying to happen.

I'm grateful to have a partner who calls me on my stuff and tells me if I'm deluding myself or side-stepping something bigger in me that's trying to emerge. It's so easy to justify my fears and emotions—to keep confirming my limited view of what's possible and to keep myself from realizing my greater potential. The only way to free myself from the constraints of our irradiated world is to recognize my self-imposed limitations and embrace the power that I have to override it all.

There's a subtle peace that envelops us as we allow these thoughts to sink in. In just a few days, we've gone from feeling huge disappointment and a deep resistance to being here, to a kind of acceptance and an openness to some higher purpose.

"Lewis?"

"Yes, wifelet?"

"Let's decide to be happy, no matter what. Let's not be a reaction to what others do or to any of this stuff coming at us. Let's choose to be happy and to define ourselves on our own terms."

"I like that idea, and there's absolutely no reason why we can't do that ... apart from the decades of negative programming about life being a struggle..."

...which, of course, is exactly what we are being challenged to change—and we're doing it.

In these conversations, I catch glimpses of anything being possible. And these probing questions always lead to others. *What changes and what becomes possible if I see the world as a safe, exciting place, rather than the unsafe, scary place it appears to be, due to all the radiation? Where would I be now—and who would I be—if that reality of a safe, exciting world had been cultivated in me from an early age?*

"Interesting questions," Lewis says, "—the kind of questions *everyone* should be asking themselves, whether they're electro-sensitive or not."

34 Becoming self-determined

Wildfires are raging across the interior of BC, covering areas the size of Ireland, with many thousands of hectares being affected. Ash fills the air, coating every surface. Technically, we're all smokers now. We can smell and see the smoke, which has blocked out the sun and the mountains in the near distance, even though the nearest fire is about 50km away. But that's not very far if you've got high winds and tinder-dry conditions, as we've been having here. We're keeping track of developments, regularly checking the fire alerts online and feeling rather vulnerable as we've never had to deal with this kind of thing before. (Did I mention that I prefer living on the coast?) We're certainly being challenged in new ways and being called upon to hone our survival skills as we prepare for a possible evacuation.

Could our situation be any more ironic? Having left behind a relatively stable environment in search of greater health and safety, we're now facing a far greater threat to our survival, in the form of these wildfires—and all our exit routes have been cut off. It was only days after we had consciously *chosen* to stay on here that all the main roads were closed, due to the fires, and leaving became impossible.

I can't help feeling that the universe is messing with me. *How bad does it have to get, Olga, before living back in that toxic EMF world seems preferable to this?* But that's just my own cynical mind talking. I know that universal intelligence doesn't work like that, and any kind of message is likely to be a lot more constructive and benevolent. Perhaps we're being pushed even deeper into survival mode so we really get to see what this is all about. Or perhaps we're being pushed deeper into ourselves and being forced to tap into our own inner resources to summon the strength and wisdom for dealing with this situation.

How do we transform this seemingly negative situation into a mechanism for moving forward? I've always believed that the key to the next step is hidden wherever you are, and that fully embracing that current place is part of what takes you onwards. On the other hand, I'm sick of this search for meaning. Most days, I'm positively happy and determined to turn this situation into a blessing. Some days, though, I feel myself dissolving into a puddle of despair.

Perhaps that's part of the process—the alternating agony and ecstasy of letting go of the old self.

Lewis has some interesting observations that distract me and get me thinking more positively again.

"It seems to me that the baggage many of us carry can find a perfect home in EHS—and a means for it to be expressed," he says, and I can see how this might be so.

I think of how I grew up never feeling safe. My home was safe and my parents were wonderful providers for us, taking care of us, celebrating our birthdays and making sure we got a good education, yet I never felt *emotionally* safe. I can see how this has translated into physical safety issues, with EMFs presenting the perfect justification for my subconscious belief that the world is not a safe place (and my first document on electromagnetic radiation was called *No Safe Place*). Strangely, I've always felt safe when in other supposedly risky situations—exploring the Amazonian jungle, being in downtown Vancouver alone at night, or travelling around the world on my own.

In the many workshops I attended in Vancouver as I learned about personal development and various healing modalities, there were group hugs and lots of emotional venting. Even though I had my own share of emotional meltdowns, I resisted this loss of control and held on tightly to my inner feelings. I preferred to stay safe and contained inside my head, where I lived for most of the time. Somehow, this need for safety got handed down through the generations, with the original source of that vulnerability lost in the multiple dramas of life. I remember my Dad telling me that his Mum (my Gran, with whom I was very close) used to hide under the bed when certain visitors came to the door. And it wasn't the tax man she was hiding from, either. She simply had an irrational fear of certain people or certain kinds of engagement.

I can relate. Even as I dreamed of being a film actress (the only thing I ever really wanted to be, growing up), and even as I became an empowerment coach and author who was called upon to do interviews and seminars, I was terrified of public speaking. I knew my fears were irrational and that they had to be addressed, so I forced myself to do workshops and other events, even though it often felt like facing a firing squad. With time, and with my work, I realized that I had been attracting the perfect people and situations to trigger my insecurities so that I could resolve them. As I did the work of facing down my fears and replacing them with self-acceptance and reassurance, I began to see magic happen in my life. My work took off. I was interviewed on breakfast TV and on radio, I did book-signing events, my client base increased rapidly (with almost no effort on my part) and money flowed into my life. As I went deeper into the healing process, however, I also attracted bigger challenges—which, I knew, were designed to take me to a higher level of awareness and empowerment, as only those bigger challenges could do.

I was really starting to clean up my act. I imagined myself going through a nice warm eco-friendly cycle in a washing machine, coming out all squeaky-clean and refreshed. Then the tumour hit, hot on the heels of my rising concerns about the microwave radiation in our environment. The trauma of this event threw me off course, even though a part of me knew that it was an even bigger challenge designed to take me to an even deeper level of awareness and empowerment. I lost my grip on the deeper truth and got caught up in fear and drama. Forget the eco-friendly wash. I was flung into an aggressive industrial washing machine and taken through the deep-dirt program. After a thorough wringing-out, I came out of the spin cycle bedraggled, dizzy and unable to get my bearings for several years. Yet the spin goes on …in government, in industry and inside ourselves.

Clearly, my fear of not being safe was so deep that an even greater challenge was required to put me in touch with some deeper subconscious layers, and it continued to have a stranglehold over my existence, despite all my conscious efforts. My sensitivity to EMFs was one expression of this, although the sensitivity was also a blessing, enabling me to facilitate the transformations of others, even if I was initially unable to facilitate my own, in the early years of my practice. Not surprisingly, given how the universe works, my fear of not being safe escalated from the personal to the planetary, with the entire microwaved world becoming an 'unsafe' place for me to be. As I worked through the layers, I realized that a fear of not being safe is really a fear of being powerful—our natural state, which has been covered up with layers of conditioning that sends us scuttling in the other direction.

**Yet the spin goes on…
in government, in industry and inside ourselves.**

Our emotional baggage manifests in all kinds of ways, with some people experiencing illness, some having career issues, and others having personal crises—all of which will take them on their own particular journey of self-discovery and healing …or not. I can see how being electro-sensitive has taken my fears to the ultimate level. Now, nowhere is safe. The radiation is real and it is everywhere. I have all the physical evidence I could possibly need to justify my reality, and my mind has lots of scientifically sound arguments to back it up. After all, it's not just me. Babies are affected, and they're not subconsciously attracting harm. Plants and animals are affected, too. So the environment needs to change, if we are to survive. It's an open-and-shut case.

"I think the only way for us to change our reality is with meditation," Lewis tells me. "We don't really believe that we can change our mindset just by choosing to believe something else. It doesn't make logical sense and you can get stuck in all the scientific evidence of harm being caused. Yet I'm convinced that changing your own reality, *despite* all that evidence, will reduce the sensitivity."

This can be difficult to embrace and I feel myself resisting. The idea of being sensitive implies that *we're* the problem. *If you weren't so sensitive, you could live a normal life*—just like other people who appear to be unaffected by what's in our environment. Yet it's not really about not being sensitive; it's about being stronger than our environment, stronger than our minds and stronger than whatever external threat might come our way.

I can think of people who had seemingly well-rounded, normal, balanced lives, only to suddenly become ill when a smart meter was installed in their home. They didn't seem to have deep emotional issues that needed to be resolved or that came to a head as a result of this external trigger. Yet that crisis will have served some purpose for them—perhaps strengthening their voice, causing a shift in their priorities, launching them on a new career path, or maybe just resulting in better self-care. Of course, there are also those who have died as a result of over-exposure, adding to the many tragedies associated with EMFs. In terms of healing myself, however, I must focus on what my reality has become. That doesn't mean that I don't care about anyone else or that we shouldn't work together to create a healthier world. It means that I can only control and change my own reality (which I have a responsibility to do) and using or relating to their reality doesn't help me to do that.

"I've noticed a vulnerability in many electro-sensitive people," Lewis says. "But is it *because* of the sensitivity or does that inner vulnerability feed the electro-sensitivity or undermine their sense of self and their power?"

"Maybe it doesn't matter," I say. "Whatever creates that vulnerability—whether it's EMFs or being abused or something else—is still a push towards greater mastery of the self."

I think about going back into the world, with all its cell towers, WiFi and uninformed consumers, and it's a scary thought. Obviously, I don't yet feel stronger than my environment or ready to tackle whatever's out there. When I contemplate returning to a more spiritual community, however, I wonder if having access to that kind of community would help me become stronger—or would all the EMFs in those community/yoga centres prevent me from even accessing that kind of support? If I forced myself to endure the radiation, would I ultimately benefit from the spiritual connection? Or is that inhospitable environment pushing me to reconnect with my own spiritual self, without any external props or support?

I can see how readily we look to others to fix things and to help us deal with stuff, while reflecting back to us the wobbly aspects of ourselves that are seeking comfort. And that's okay. We all need support. The challenge is knowing when it's healthy support and when it's a kind of dependence and a way to stay stuck. Our minds can keep us distracted forever with their logic, pre-programmed beliefs and fear-based projections.

I have several close friends who are deeply spiritual and who seem to be impervious to all the man-made radiation. Through meditation, yoga, chanting and movement/dance, they have expanded their own chi and their own electromagnetic field to the point that they are stronger than the EMFs coming at them from outside. Music is something else that seems to feature prominently in the lives of those who are healthy and have a strong resilience to EMFs. The musicians I know have a very strong core. They also seem to be very calm, grounded, open and present. This is a missing element in my life and one that I have let slip away, without realizing it. Doesn't take a rocket scientist to figure out what I need to do about that.

Being passionately engaged in your work, exercising vigorously every day, playing music, breathing deeply, meditating and enjoying friendship and laughter with like-minded individuals seems like the natural antidote to many of life's challenges—including electro-sensitivity. If I can engage in all of those things, while in this healthy low-EMF environment, I can't imagine not emerging a great deal stronger.

Disengaging from the irradiated world is not enough on its own without all these other elements. Isolating myself won't bring about that kind of holistic healing or overall strengthening of my system. In a sense, by retreating, I've become almost two-dimensional, when I really need to be multi-dimensional. I must take myself to a higher dimension in order to protect myself from what seems insanely inhuman and physically insurmountable. I don't want to be backed into a corner, in a state of retreat; I want to *expand* my whole being to the point where I'm having a positive outward effect rather than being diminished by, or at the effect of, something imposed on me from the outside.

"We don't want to be depending on our environment to make us feel okay," says Lewis. "We want to command it. And if we have a strong enough core, we can have more of an effect on things while being less affected by them."

After being here for almost six weeks, I see that I must use this relative isolation as an opportunity to become stronger on every level and to be far more than I was, before being affected by EMFs. While there is huge value in stripping away all the external distractions and stimulation in that multi-tasking, always-on, addictively connected world, it won't count for much unless I incorporate these various pillars of regeneration to create a much more resilient holistic self. Having a more balanced, joyous, dynamic, musical, engaging and spiritually nourishing lifestyle is essential to creating that solid foundation.

"I think it's important for you to just *experience* those things and to stop trying to figure things out," says Lewis, who knows all too well how my overly analytical mind can get in the way. Making sense of things, always looking for reasons, and coming up with great ideas—none of it means anything unless it translates into action.

So I took action. Every morning, I did some yoga and Qigong to wake up my body. I mowed the grass using our manual lawnmower, which is a bit misleading as the *lawn* is more like a field, although you could practically play golf on it when I'd finished. I meditated for at least an hour every afternoon and then I did some writing. I bounced about 400 times on the trampoline, shaking it all up. In the evening, I played table tennis with my man. We were both surprisingly good, neither of us having played for decades, yet we still managed to laugh ourselves silly when we played, which was exactly what we needed after so much seriousness.

After a week of this, I feel calmer and more connected to myself. I experience periods of contentment and a quiet kind of peace. I trust that things will work out positively and that it's all taken care of. Working my body, feeding my spirit and getting my mind out of the way seems to be the way to go.

35 Remembering who we are

In grappling with health challenges and the dangers of electromagnetic radiation—all seemingly *serious* stuff—it occurs to me that I've never really *enjoyed* life. I enjoy my work and I've experienced many wonderful breakthroughs, joyous occasions, exciting adventures and heartfelt connections, but I don't think I've embraced enjoyment as a lifestyle or a philosophy to live by. Yet that is what life is all about—enjoying ourselves and enjoying *being* ourselves. The human body is designed for enjoyment and pleasure, having the senses, sensuality and sexuality to feel things on many levels—and to be transported beyond the physical, to experience ecstasy, love and a spiritual connection. To exist largely in the material world, as avid consumers caught up in the physical gratification we get from money, success and the power of our high-tech gadgets, seems very limiting, given our multi-dimensional nature.

If we focused on being all that we could be, while loving and living that, how might we be different? If we looked at every experience and opportunity in terms of how much joy it could give us and others, how would that affect our choices and their outcomes? How would our relationships be affected if we only engaged in interactions and business dealings that were positively uplifting? If joy set the tone and context for our lives, how powerful would we be? When we fall in love and experience that effervescent vibrancy and the heady sense of everything being possible, we get a sense of how much power resides inside us. It's similar to what we feel when we tap into universal consciousness and experience the magic of being able to manifest what we envision.

I have experienced this—being in the flow and having things effortlessly and magically fall into place. It's natural to love life when you're in this state because life seems to love you right back. And the more you embrace this way of living, the more love and magic you experience. There was a period in my life when I was deeply spiritual and had a telepathic connection with my partner at the time. I felt powerfully alive, tuned in to the universe and very much loved and cared for by it. I never worried about money or having clients, and I never had a shortage of either one. Yet, along the way, my heart got hurt and it shut down—and my spirit, in solidarity, decided to

162

also go on strike. It's as if it became a soul-satellite, orbiting my body, while I fumbled along without it, resorting to my mental prowess to pick up the slack. My focus switched from experiencing a deep, nourishing connection, to analysing what was going on outside me and why. Without consciously realizing it, I went from a state of relative mastery over my circumstances, to being vulnerable to attack. The stage was set for harm to set in and for that vulnerability to manifest in physical form.

I know how powerful we are when we are spiritually attuned, but I lost sight of all that when the effects of electro-sensitivity hit home. I forgot who I was, how I operated and what I was capable of, and I got lost in being a victim. I allowed myself to be distracted by all the neurological symptoms and then, unimaginably, a brain tumour. Instead of seeing it for what it was—a call back to wholeness, a reminder of the imbalance in my life—I sank further into the spiritual disconnect and relied even more heavily on my mind to try to understand and fix things. And here I am, over a decade later, picking up the all-important pieces of me that got marginalized and abandoned along the way. If I can once again be fuelled by that love of self and life, and tuned in to universal intelligence and my own soul's wisdom, I can regain that sense of indomitability. There is very little we cannot do if we are in touch with our soul and powered by joy, love and a passion for life.

In the context of healing from the impact of EMFs (or anything else), I believe that enjoyment and pleasure are key qualities to be embraced. To experience either of these things, we must be emotionally connected. And if our unique electromagnetic signature is determined by what we think and feel, how much more resilient and powerful would it be if it were filled with joyous energy, without the weighty, depleting effect of fears, insecurities or self-doubt?

But how do you develop a *hunger* for enjoyment? From a place of illness, exhaustion or defeat about life and its apparent EMF-imposed limits, how do you savour life and live it to the fullest? How do you develop an excitement for new experiences, travel to new places and interactions with new people … when they all seem to present a threat?

For many electro-sensitive people, it can seem impossible to regain that zest for life—if they ever had it. Ironically, it's the insensitivity of the majority that often leads to the super-sensitivity of the few, creating a strong duality of opposites. This reminds me of a principle in psychology in the context of relationships: if one partner suppresses his/her anger, the other partner may end up expressing it instead.

Many of us are at the opposite end of the spectrum of what's healthy, experiencing our own conflicting dualities inside. Fear and dread are at one end, love and joy at the other.

I don't want to stay stuck in that mode of vulnerability. I want to be at the other end of the spectrum, loving life and living it fearlessly, with passion, real enthusiasm and positive expectations.

Given where I am now, what would that take? Being grateful for what is and for what I envision for the future. Loving what *is* creates more of the same. I find joy in watching the hummingbirds guzzling the sugared water from the feeder outside our dining-room window. I can't help smiling as they zoom around, chasing any other hummers that come near their precious food, even though there are four 'watering holes', with plenty for everyone. I watch as one guzzles the sweet liquid, sending bubbles up the glass jar, and then freezes when another bird lands on the other side of the feeder. I can almost feel it glaring and sending out buzz-off vibes. *Hey, pal. This is MY feeder. Am I invisible or what? Okay, that's it.* And it chases the other hummingbird away.

I feel an almost overwhelming tenderness for the little fluffy ball of a bird that seems to enjoy resting on our doorstep every morning. It shows no fear and just looks up at us, cocking its head from side to side, as we walk by. *Yes? You want something? Can't you see I'm trying to relax, here?* Yet it's not injured and will eventually fly off in search of whatever other bliss it can find in nature. No ruffled feathers or even fear where it would seem to be justified, which seems to offer a profound metaphor for frazzled humans.

I can even enjoy the deep-throated lowing of the free-ranging cattle in the area, which often wander onto the property. When they appear one day inside the fenced-off area around the house, I can't figure out how they got in. The fence seems to be intact, yet there they are—three heifers nonchalantly chomping on the grass, while the grown-ups watch from the other side, unfazed by this brazenness. After watching for a few minutes, I shoo them off …and they calmly jump the three-foot fence from a standing start. I had no idea cattle could jump like that. *Yeah. That's the way we roll. Coolest bovines in the hood.*

When you stop to commune with nature, you realize that everything out there speaks to you. It's easy to love animals when they're so committed to being what they are, minding their own business and just doing their own thing, without harming anyone else. If only humans could be that committed to being fully human, while happily co-existing with each other and reveling in self-mastery.

I think of the resentment, judgement and anger I have felt when I encountered someone with a cell phone or wireless device. I saw them as a source of harm, a confirmation of me not being important, the embodiment of a violated boundary and a lack of respect. I have no doubt that those intensely negative feelings did me just as much harm as the radiation itself— if not more. And they were all of my own making. If I truly want to fortify my body so that it is unaffected by these ambient EMFs, I must transform those old reactions into a love for the humans involved and for humanity itself. After all, isn't that what this is all about—trying to restore a healthy balance in our world so we can live the kind of inspired, fulfilling lives we're capable of living? I can see these interactions as an opportunity for me to love life—by loving *them*, instead of focusing on the potential harm they could do me. I can choose to be bigger and stronger than that. I will not let a cell phone run my life—even if they let it run theirs, albeit in an entirely different way.

Also essential to regaining my *joie de vivre* is a healthy sense of entitlement—a deep recognition of my right to exist and to thrive, in safety and good health. I have a friend who has an interesting perspective on this. Having rid herself of cancer, overcome other significant challenges, informed herself about EMR, created her own healthy living environment, successfully fought off encroaching cell towers in her neighbourhood, and very purposefully mastered herself on many levels, she has tremendous physical, emotional and spiritual strength. From this perspective of healthy self-determination, she can see beneath the superficial layers of reality that most people accept without question.

"Nearly every well-meaning source expressing EMF concerns seems to do so in a way that actually supports resistance to change," she says. "It promotes impotence to change and fear about what is happening."

This fits with my active quest for joy and contentment, while letting go of the fear that has run my life for far too long. Having worked with hundreds of clients for over two decades, connecting with them on a very real, heartfelt level, it's strange to now find myself feeling a need to regain my love for life.

"It takes an inward force to counter an artificial force," she says, which echoes the principles of quantum physics that I've been working with. "Why are so many willing to remain such supplicants—so compliant with sickness, disease and death?"

My friend also introduced me to the practice of Chi Lel[71]—a powerful form of meditation designed to heal illness and emotional angst. She shared the story of a friend with breast cancer who was exposed to deadly levels of radiation yet was able to protect herself from any ill-effects by doing Chi Lel.

But even to talk about *healing*, she says, implies that we are somehow flawed or in need of fixing. She refuses to use that term with herself, preferring instead to focus on solutions. "Too many people obsess about the problem," she says, "almost as if they have an addiction to suffering."

Any analysis that ignores solutions is incomplete and part of the problem, she adds, only serving to promote a sense of helplessness, impotence and paralysis. I know that the real breakthroughs come from strengthening our own power, rather than endlessly appealing to the authorities to please listen to us and protect us. Appealing to the authorities to help us actually empowers them while disempowering us.

"In focusing on those who are behind the proliferation of microwave technologies, too many people remain transfixed like a mongoose hypnotized by a cobra," says my friend, whose feistiness always makes me smile. "I'm weary of listening to those who remain problem-oriented but do not evolve or move forward towards being solution-oriented."

Decades ago, working with a martial arts friend, she used to teach self-defence to women who had been abused or attacked.

"What is *wrong* with these women?" her friend asked. "Where is their sense of entitlement to retaliate, to defend themselves effectively, to defeat the opponent or the attacker? Why do I feel such a wall of resignation and passivity—the absence of any useful directed anger or any sense of indignation? Where is their assuredness that they possess the right to not be assaulted and, more to the point, to fight back and win?"

This lack of healthy entitlement seems to be a big part of the problem in dealing with EMFs. Unless we actively embrace that sense of entitlement in our lives and claim our right to thrive and live freely, without harm, we will remain at the mercy of those who feel more entitled than we do.

"We are inherently powerful energy creatures," my friend says, "yet too many see themselves as vulnerable and weak, which becomes a self-fulfilling prophecy. Think weak, stay weak. But why do so many succumb before their time—to EHS, cancer or whatever—rather than choosing to change? It's as if fear of change is greater than fear of dying …and maybe it is, for some. And that is my definition of enslavement. *Pulling on chains is not breaking them.*"

Hard-won wisdom from someone who has surmounted her own significant health challenges with electromagnetic radiation and has emerged victorious, healthy and whole. She has walked the talk and is still walking it, with little tolerance for self-pity. She raises other important questions that we might benefit from asking ourselves if we truly want to have a life worth living: *What stops us from self-love and self-nurturance? Why do we not choose to eat well and strengthen our bodies so we can overcome frequency susceptibility? Do we not care for ourselves enough to daily practise the self-loving, self-respecting, feel-good processes that heal and put a protective shield in place—a shield of our own making, using our minds and a strong electromagnetic field?*

The answers to these questions, if truthfully and diligently explored, can take us on a journey of self-awareness, away from a dependence on those who have failed to do what is right, and towards a solid reliance on the inner forces that we must activate to become truly self-sufficient and empowered. This is autonomy—the individual sovereignty that each of us can claim, without the help, support or permission of the so-called authorities. This is what makes us safe, strong and resilient, operating at a far higher level than our supposed leaders. If we dig deeply into our spiritual, emotional and neurological prowess, and if we invest our resources into being fully, powerfully ourselves, rather than squandering them on the fight against those who harm us, we can make ourselves invulnerable.

The very best gift we can give ourselves and each other, then, is to remember and embody who we really are, how life really works and what our challenges represent, beyond their physical impact.

36 Relating, bonding, belonging: we are hard-wired to connect

Imagine living a life of total solitude, without any interaction with other human beings. Would you have any idea of who you were? And how much fun, meaning and enjoyment would you have if you were totally alone?

We are born to interact and connect with others, and it is our relationships that make our lives meaningful. Without human interaction, nothing much would happen and we would feel emotionally empty and malnourished. We know that infants need human touch and affection in order to thrive, so it should not surprise us that adults need the same emotional bonds and reassurance. We also need other people in our lives to show us who we are and who we can become. Without those sounding boards and mirrors of our deeper selves, we would have no one to react to, collaborate with, inspire, be jealous of, encourage, support or love. We would have no means of experiencing the full range of human emotions, as triggered or nourished by those around us. Whether we are relating to our partner, employer, friend or enemy, we are always in some form of relationship. And *how* we relate to the world determines how it relates back to us. The solutions to our conflicts with others—be they individuals or large corporations—come from understanding and resolving our inner conflicts, and relationships provide the key to this journey of discovery, healing and evolution.

**How we relate to the world
determines how it relates back to us.**

As physical beings with an electromagnetic field and a highly developed central nervous system, we are broadcasting and receiving information every moment of our existence. Our electrical field and cellular memory are filled with electrical and emotional charges relating to our life experiences, and they tell their own story independently of our verbal communication. This communication network is in constant interaction with the outside world,

168

reacting to stimuli, filtering information, and generally acting as a radar system for our physical selves. And it's no accident that we are physiologically 'wired' to connect with others, since this primal instinct is fundamental to our fulfillment as human beings.

As a relationship therapist (and from personal experience), I know how pivotal relationships are to our well-being, growth and happiness. Whether we like to admit it or not, we want and need to be loved. We are social beings with a built-in need for connection and a sense of belonging—two qualities that may be missing from the lives of those who are electro-sensitive, due to the isolation they often experience. While the massive explosion of social media interaction shows us just how strong is our need to connect, this kind of connection rarely meets that need in a meaningful way. Emojis, likes and shares won't give you the same warm fuzzy feelings as a close personal contact, and you can't hug your friends on Facebook. Although many deep connections are made online, much of this social interaction is about distraction, stimulation and a striving to belong. The kind of meaningful connection we seek goes much deeper.

The social media connections I have made that are meaningful are those that have developed into real friendships, with phone calls, personal exchanges and heartfelt sharing. No longer just a name or a Facebook friend, they are real people with lives and feelings that matter to me.

We all want love in its many forms: acceptance, support, validation, encouragement and respect. If we claim otherwise, it's usually because we have been hurt or rejected, which leads us to believe that we are unlovable or unworthy. But love is not only absolutely possible for all; it's our birthright and the greatest human imperative.

"Our need to connect is as fundamental as our need for food and water" says scientist Matthew Lieberman, author of Social, which explores the neuroscience of human connections.[72] Based on the data, he says, it is clear that "we are profoundly shaped by our social environment and that we suffer greatly when our social bonds are threatened or severed. When this happens in childhood it can lead to long-term health and educational problems. We may not like the fact that […] our well-being depends on our connections with others, but the facts are the facts."

Social pain can cause real, physical pain, which is why we so often try to fit in, be liked and be accepted. Being wired this way is both a blessing and a curse. On the one hand, it "helps to ensure that we'll have the same kind of beliefs and values as those of the people around us and this is a great catalyst for social harmony," says Lieberman. On the other hand, it means that we may readily compromise our own beliefs and values in order to be liked/loved.

Our need for meaningful connection has a very real impact on our health, creating stress and many serious conditions. "Being alone can literally break your heart," says Ray Hainer, who documents how this chronic form of stress can lead to heart disease.[73] Research shows that those who lack a strong network of friends and family are at greater risk of developing and dying from heart disease.

In recent years, says Hainer, researchers have begun to unravel the cardiovascular effects of social isolation, and they've discovered that *feeling* alone may hurt the heart even more than actually *being* alone. Since the heart plays such a fundamental role in our well-being, being socially/emotionally isolated makes us more susceptible to all forms of disease.

Emotional alienation is exactly what's happening to electro-sensitive individuals who have retreated into the sidelines because of the impact of electromagnetic radiation. This places an additional burden on their hearts, beyond the adverse effects of EMR exposure. Yet we have all been alienated to some degree, whether it's by the wireless telecoms industry, uncaring governments, schoolyard bullies or due to the loss/rejection of a loved one.

Yet the very thing that we so desperately strive to create, through non-stop mobile connectivity, is the very thing that is disconnecting us from our natural instincts of caring, sharing and community collaboration. We cannot truly care unless we have a meaningful connection with someone. Only then will they care about us or our situation. I have seen this happen many times, in the context of dealing with EMFs, although it is true for all areas of life. Trying to convey the dangers of microwave radiation to someone who doesn't know you rarely works. But if you develop a relationship with them, they are far more open to hearing what you have to say …and to believing you.

If we choose convenience over health, we cannot claim to care. And this impersonal stance is a direct reflection of our lack of emotional connection to those who are affected by our indifference. It is up to us, therefore, to cultivate more meaningful connections in our lives—for the sake of our own well-being and for the well-being of our planet.

**If we choose convenience over health,
we cannot claim to care.**

We may not even realize that our hearts have shut down or gone into overload, until or unless we make a profoundly meaningful, loving connection with another. We may be multi-tasking and moving so fast, flitting from one thing to another and getting stuck in the past while worrying about the future, that we are completely disconnected from ourselves and our behaviour. Only by connecting with others in a heartfelt way will we understand what we have been missing. Only by healing and deepening our relationships will we care about what we do to each other and to the planet. Without that emotional investment, we're far less likely to care and we'll tend to treat each other and our world as a commodity to be exploited for our personal pleasure and convenience.

Healing our relationship with self and, by extension, with others, will help to heal our emotionally fragmented selves, our physically impacted bodies and our addicted brains. Cultivating loving relationships is the key to fortifying our bodies and minds, whether we're grappling with the effects of EMFs or problems with a partner. We all need each other, and we exist together, on this planet, so that we can learn how to relate, interact, love, evolve and co-create in harmony, to the benefit of all.

When we work together, we are stronger and our brains start to become neurologically entrained, scientists confirm.[74] Our brain waves become synchronised when, as a group, we focus or work on the same thing. This makes us much more powerful than the sum of our separate parts.

We can apply this concept collectively, to address the invasive EMFs in our lives. Nature is on our side. Our brains and bodies are ready and willing to serve us. We just need to understand how they operate and how to give our hearts and souls the meaningful emotional connections that they need in order to build resilience, thrive and restore balance in our world.

"We urgently need to find practical ways of reestablishing our conscious sense of connection with living nature."

—Rupert Sheldrake, in *The Rebirth of Nature*

37 Addiction: the real reason for our denial

Many people now spend more time in the virtual world than the real one, unaware of the repercussions for our humanity and our natural environment. Yet many of us are aware that something is seriously wrong with the way we are living. Even those who are not electro-sensitive are seeing and feeling the impacts of social fragmentation, too much screen time and not enough loving human interaction. Yet no amount of compelling evidence and wisdom will change this reality if addiction is the underlying cause. And the addiction to social media and mobile connectivity is now so pervasive and so deeply entrenched that it is hard to see how it might ever be addressed.

When you realize that social media megaliths such as Facebook are designed to intentionally hook consumers in a very real way, you begin to understand just how far down this digital rabbit hole we have gone. In the same way that many processed foods are designed to be addictive, we are being deliberately manipulated into becoming physically and emotionally dependent on the social media networks that are touted to enhance our lives in countless ways (see box). In reality, they have hijacked our hearts and our humanity, while promoting non-stop wireless connectivity.

As a society, we have sold our souls to the social-media moguls and have become pawns in their algorithmically manipulated games. They can sell us anything—and they do, peddling the promise of eternal entertainment, rewards, happiness and redemption.

Algorithmically yours...

As Eric Andrew-Gee reports in *The Globe and Mail* in January 2018,[75] ex-president of Facebook, Sean Parker, recently admitted that the social media platform was designed to hook users with spurts of dopamine—the neurotransmitter released when the brain expects a reward or acquires fresh knowledge. "You're exploiting a vulnerability in human psychology," he said. "[The inventors] understood this, consciously, and we did it anyway."

Now, says Andrew-Gee, some of the early executives of these tech firms consider their success to be tainted:

Chamath Palihapitiya, former vice-president of user growth at Facebook, said he felt tremendous guilt. "I think we all knew in the back of our minds... something bad could happen. [...] The short-term, dopamine-driven feedback loops that we have created are destroying how society works [and] eroding the core foundations of how people behave."

Tristan Harris, a former Google product manager, now leads an initiative to wean consumers off the attention-destroying technology he helped create. "Smartphones are 'literally using the power of billion-dollar computers to figure out what to feed you [...] That's why you can't look away.'" Sophisticated algorithms are used to send us targeted messages and emotional hooks, tailored to our needs and designed to grab our attention. But, Harris says, "We're going to look back and say, 'Why on earth did we do this?'"

A decade into this age of connectedness, we have learned something troubling, says Andrew-Gee. "Being connected to everyone all the time makes us less attentive to the people we care about most. Nowhere is the alienating power of smartphones more troubling than in the relationship between parents and children. Put simply, smartphones are making mothers and fathers pay less attention to their kids and it could be causing emotional harm."

> "We still haven't understood or accepted how completely smartphones have distorted [...] our relationships with ourselves and with the reality around us. We are divorced from ourselves and from the world."[76]
> —Lev Grossman, *Time* magazine technology writer

In the process, we have lost an essential part of ourselves, and we are now stuck in a loop, addicted to a technology that is taking us further and further away from what we need most, while deepening our dependence and our emotional disconnect.

"Humans long to feel connected," says Alison Main, in Addicted to iLove: the consequences of connected reality (*Paleo* magazine).[77] "We leave our cribs and our plush toys, but we still cling to a security blanket—and now this one is addictively glowing. There's no other invention that has ever hit the spot so accurately, appeasing our innate fears of isolation and disconnection. With our digital technologies, we can be alone but never alone. [And] we are together, but never together. Unfortunately, we have tethered our humanity to something without a biological pulse."

Less connection—the real kind—means that families aren't able to build relationships as strong as they could be, says Jim Taylor, PhD, in *Psychology Today*.[78] Nor are they able to maintain them as well. As a result, children will feel less familiarity, comfort, trust, security and, most importantly, love from their parents.

We all have connection issues, but going wireless 24/7 will not resolve them.

Ironically, it is our deep human need for connection that has led us to depend on forms of communication that provide momentary pleasure, yet prevent us from connecting in heartfelt, nourishing ways ...while exposing us to harmful radiation.

Addiction has less to do with the pleasurable effects of substances, claims journalist Johann Hari, than with the user's inability to connect in healthy ways with other human beings. In other words, addiction is not a substance disorder; *it is a social disorder*.[79] While this might seem simplistic, it makes sense, since most human dysfunction comes from an unmet need for love, acceptance, emotional connection and validation of who we are. We can see the impact of this loss of connection all around us, and the addiction to perpetual mobile connectivity is the inevitable manifestation of this missing human element.

"The opposite of addiction is connection," says author and relationship expert Robert Weiss.[80] The human need for trust and attachment was initially studied in the 1950s by John Bowlby, who found that infants, toddlers and young children have an extensive need for safe and reliable caregivers. "If children have that," says Weiss, "they tend to be happy in childhood and well-adjusted (emotionally healthy) later in life. If children don't have that, it's a very different story." Research has shown that those who experience secure attachment as infants, toddlers and small children can naturally trust and connect in healthy ways, says Weiss. Those who don't experience secure early-life attachment tend to struggle with trust and connection later in life. "Guess which group is more vulnerable to addiction."

With human addicts, the recovery process nearly always involves overcoming the lack of trust and connection created in childhood, says Weiss ...which is what we are now being challenged to do if we want to have healthy relationships in a healthy world.

The cycle of harm... and how to break it

By nature, we are caring, loving beings, but our capacity for compassion and emotional availability has been suppressed—and is further diminished by exposure to microwave radiation. Due to emotional neglect, negative experiences or loss in our early years, we have switched off parts of ourselves to disconnect from our pain so that we can function.

Pain and love live together in our hearts. They take turns at being in charge, although pain usually wins, if it's bigger. For many of us, our emotional pain is so deeply buried that we don't even know it is there. We might claim to be fine, enjoying life, working, managing... but our hearts would disagree, if given a say. We may talk about being well adjusted, but adjusted to what— not being unconditionally loved or accepted, not feeling good enough, not loving our life? We should not have to adjust to the absence of things that foster life and fulfillment.

When we are disconnected from our hearts, we are disconnected from the harm that has been done to us ...and that we have done to ourselves and our planet. We can only live in our technologically driven world if we are emotionally disconnected; and only emotionally disconnected people would create this kind of world. Disconnected from our pain and deeper feelings, we live and function dispassionately, speedily and distractedly, without realizing that our hearts have gone offline.

Having worked with hundreds of people from all walks of life, I know that every single one of them (me included) carries some pain, loss and sadness. Some of those I worked with had become so emotionally disconnected that they put all their energy into their business and improving their finances, without doing the emotional work required to ensure their success. Some felt that their pain was so huge that, if they opened up their hearts after suppressing things for so long, they would fall apart and never stop crying. But most embraced the work of healing themselves, knowing that they would never be happy or fulfilled unless they did.

Many of us are so disconnected from our feelings that we don't even know what we feel. I was almost 30 years old before I realized how unhappy I was—or that I was unhappy at all. Based on appearances, you would have thought I was doing very well: I was married, with a fabulous job, lots of friends and a privileged, affluent lifestyle in Switzerland. But I had become so good at hiding my feelings—from myself and from the world—that I didn't know what I was missing or how much of me had been suppressed.

Our denial of the dangers of electromagnetic radiation is due to our addiction to social media and mobile connectivity. Our addiction is caused by an emotional disconnect. And the emotional disconnect is caused by a shortage of early emotional nourishment (love/bonding/support/safety) that has left us feeling incomplete, needy, insecure or diminished in some way. That emotional deficit will keep us stuck forever, unless we acknowledge and address the deeper root of our dysfunction, as well as the resistance we have to taking responsibility for it. Unless we do that, the proliferation of wireless radiation in our environment is likely to continue unchecked, with most leaders and decision-makers every bit as addicted as those they are tasked with protecting.

Because we are so addicted to social media and mobile connectivity, we rationalize our constant use of a smartphone (or other wireless device) with seemingly justifiable claims: I need it for my work. It's my life—all my friends and family are online. My business depends on me being available 24/7. It saves me time and money. I feel safer and more secure with my phone on me at all times. What if there's an emergency?

The list of justifications is endless—and entirely plausible, as all addicts will agree. Most people do need an Internet connection for their work (and social media can be informative and a lot of fun), but when, where, how and how often people connect determines whether they are enhancing or diminishing their quality of life ...not to mention their health, cognitive function, memory, capacity for empathy, relationships and personal development. There is even a new term, says Main, to define the fear of being without mobile-phone contact: nomophobia.

Given the nature of addiction, however, addicts are unlikely to acknowledge their unhealthy dependence or rationally assess their behaviour. Even asking them simple questions about their needs is more likely to generate irritation and annoyance than considered, conscious reflection about what's really going on.

Do you absolutely need to be wirelessly connected around the clock? Do you need to be online during mealtime, when relaxing, when spending time with your children/spouse/friends? Must you have your smartphone beside your bed, turned on and ready for action—even if it means interrupting intimacy with a partner? Most would answer yes to all of these questions.

Relationships—and the art of relating itself—are being threatened by the mania for superficial connections. Having a smartphone in your bedroom is like having a third person in the room, creating an e-love triangle—or quadrangle, if your partner has his/hers there too. Relationships can get very crowded when there are so many parties involved. And it's hard to stay focused on the task at hand when there is always the possibility of a call, text or notification that requires your immediate attention.

Nowhere is exempt, it seems. Parks, beaches, forests and even retreat centres now all have WiFi and/or cell phone coverage. Being constantly connected to others means that we are less and less connected to ourselves and to what it means to be fully human.

"Don't sacrifice your humanity for a techno-utopia," urges Main. "Facebook doesn't love you. It only cares how much you 'Like' it" …and how much you respond to the multitude of ads, share your thoughts and feed the beast.

The devastating socio-emotional disconnection promoted by digital addiction also fosters a disconnection from our natural world, with equally devastating consequences.

We delude ourselves into believing that humans are immune to the laws of nature and can magically replenish our planet's finite resources.

"As techno-literacy expands, eco-literacy contracts," says Erica Etelson.[81] "We know how to create PowerPoint presentations, but don't know a watershed from a wetland. Worse, the more tech-savvy and eco-ignorant we become, the more we delude ourselves into believing that humans are immune to the laws of nature and can magically replenish our planet's finite resources."

The undermining of our sense of social and personal responsibility (which comes from our loss of emotional connectedness) has alarming consequences for our natural environment. "We're unwilling to take even relatively simple, easy steps that would reduce demand for water, electricity and fuel," says Etelson, "unless a smart marketing campaign convinces us that we'll save big bucks. Modern conveniences have not only made us lazy, but have led us to assume that the arc of human betterment is inevitable, and that we are but passive observers of its triumphant mastery over nature."

As electromagnetic beings, *we* are designed to radiate out into the world, not to be irradiated and cancelled out by man-made devices with no soul.

A recovering human rights attorney, an environmental activist and a writer, Etelson has identified 10 dangers of technology, including our loss of resilience in the face of everyday challenges.

"Our deluded pride in our species' intelligence blinds us to the core deception of technology—that it makes us more resilient," she says. "Evaluate your own resilience next time you turn on the faucet; what would you do if nothing came out? Do you even know where your water comes from? Many of us cannot imagine how we would survive without mobile phones, much less indoor plumbing."

As members of modern society, we think we are very clever, says Etelson, even though we lack even rudimentary knowledge of the biological and artificial life systems that support us.

"Technology separates us from the natural world by diverting our focus from natural to human-made wonders," she says. "Every day, we are offered a free gift of joy and serenity courtesy of Mother Nature, but we usually opt instead for artificial pleasures like video games. A vicious cycle is born, in which our separation from nature and from each other leaves us feeling empty and compels us to seek more creature comforts to fill the hole, and we then become addicted to the pleasure of consuming and spend even less time connecting with people and nature."

The delusion that we are separate from nature is the perilous essence of the techno-topian myth, says Etelson. And the sooner we shatter it, the better.

What will it take for us to come to our senses?

Many of us, whether electro-sensitive or not, are already painfully aware of the repercussions of digital addiction, but stacking up the evidence of harm won't cure it. Clearly, awareness of what this is costing us is not enough. We need a very good reason—and a significant payoff—for reducing our dependence on electronic gadgets and wireless connectivity. If we can acknowledge what we have lost and most want to have in life, we can start to reconnect with our deep desire and unmet need for human love and acceptance. Only when we reconnect with our hearts and deeper emotions will we begin to grasp the enormity of what we have done—to ourselves and to our planet.

Addiction inhibits awareness (which is one reason why it exists), and only conscious awareness will cure the underlying cause. Whether you are an e-addict or an electro-sensitive individual who has been affected by this global addiction, the solution is the same: a return to emotional availability, healthy self-responsibility, and a willingness to resolve your own emotional deficits in real time, with real people and with real awareness.

If you teeter on the edge, caught up in the frenzy but not yet deeply addicted, there is hope for a quick recovery. Come back to the real world, to what really matters, and to what feeds your heart and soul.

Only we can cure our own addiction, since it requires a conscious desire—and a recognition of the need—for something far more rewarding: more love, more heartfelt connection, more intimacy, more acceptance, more empathy, more community involvement, more communing with nature, more emotional honesty and more quality time with loved ones.

**Addiction inhibits awareness and
only conscious awareness will cure the underlying cause.**

All addictions yield diminishing returns, with the downsides eventually outweighing the perceived benefits ...and changing us greatly, in the process.

We must be willing to explore our motivations, to identify what's missing in our lives, and to acknowledge what drives our addiction. We must recognize our resistance to weaning ourselves off our addictive habits and devices. We must see our rationalizations for what they are, even if they seem legitimate. It's not a matter of convincing me or anyone else that you absolutely need social media or non-stop connectivity; it's about understanding what it's costing you, what you are losing, and where you will end up if you continue down this e-road. It is not a nice destination and your GPS device won't be able to guide you back home.

38 Digital descendants: our children pay the e-price

It's not just our social media addiction that affects us, and it's not just adults that are affected. The cognitive, emotional and social development of toddlers and children is also being seriously undermined by unhealthy amounts of screen time (usually on a microwave-radiation-emitting wireless device), with Electronic Screen Syndrome now a recognized disorder. The syndrome promotes a fight-or-flight response, which leads to the "dysregulation and disorganization of various biological systems," says integrative psychiatrist Dr Victoria Dunkley, MD, author of *Reset Your Child's Brain*.[82]

"The majority of neuroscientists believe that the overuse of online activity is harming children," reports Daniel Riseman, referencing recognized neurological experts.[83] "Spending hours in the virtual world has led to the deterioration in a child's ability to read people's facial expressions and understand emotional context." This, he says, has resulted in social interactions becoming more awkward, with greater misinterpretation during face-to-face meetings, promoting problems ranging from poor comprehension of classroom lessons to bullying among peers. "Children's addiction to online activity has resulted in less interaction with other kids outside of school," says Riseman, "and, according to developmental psychologist Dr Peter Gray, children who do not interact much with other kids have a higher likelihood of becoming aggressive and selfish adults." The consequences can be even more serious, Riseman notes. "The dramatic rise in school shootings may be directly connected to such isolation as these young shooters follow a gaming-like script as they ruthlessly murder their classmates."

"The facts are frightening: one in six children has a diagnosed mental illness, and aggressive and unmanageable behavior has become the norm at many schools across the country."[84]

In France and Switzerland, doctors and teachers are also sounding the alarm about children's over-exposure to digital devices, reports Sophie Davaris.[85] "Pediatricians and child psychiatrists, psychologists, speech and language pathologists raised a 'major public health issue'," says Davaris, referring to an article in *Le Monde*. "Overexposure to digital technology causes a host of ailments. Whatever the social environment, these specialists describe children who are not developing normally: they do not speak, they do not communicate, they are very agitated or, conversely, they are passive. According to the authors, these disorders are similar to the symptoms of autism, with the major difference that they disappear when screens are removed."

In Geneva, Davaris says, child psychiatrist Nathalie Nanzer, deputy physician in charge of the Child Guidance Unit at Geneva's university hospital (HUG), highlights the danger of screens for toddlers. "Faced with screens before the age of 1, children experience great developmental delays," says Nanzer. "Towards age 2–3, hyperactive and disorganized, they cannot concentrate. At age 3–4, some children are without language and without interaction. They do not look at you, do not know how to say hello or to ask for something from their mother." These are toddlers who are awkward in their walking and gestures. "Some have never held a pencil! They do not know how to play Lego, they get upset and send everything flying."

How will these children behave, 10 or 20 years from now? What kind of friendships and relationships will they have, and how will these early mental-health and cognitive issues play out, later in life? How will they survive in the world of business? Will they be emotionally or mentally self-sufficient as adults? Would *you* want to be married to someone like this?

The damage caused by over-use of digital devices is compounded by the WiFi that usually enables those devices. Knowing how microwave radiation affects my brain, causing dizziness, disorientation and foggy thinking, I can imagine the impact it must be having on children exposed to it in schools … not just diminishing their cognitive function, memory and concentration, but also making it very hard for them to think straight and process basic information. How many of these children are labelled as having Attention Deficit Disorder (ADD) or as being *slow* or *mentally challenged* when, in reality, their vulnerable young brains are being scrambled by microwaves?

The damage is often far more serious than that, as atomic physicist and microwave-radiation expert, Barrie Trower, so compellingly explains. With a degree in nuclear and atomic physics and microwave absorption, a second degree in the environmental influence on thinking processes, and a teaching diploma in human physiology, Barrie has a unique understanding of the biological effects of microwave radiation. He also studied microwave warfare when he worked as an underwater bomb disposal diver in the 1960s with the Royal Navy, which used microwaves as a weapon—and *it is the perfect stealth weapon*, he says. When he left the Navy, he spent 11 years questioning captured Russian spies involved in microwave warfare against the Americans, learning even more about how these microwaves could be used to ill effect.

"There is no safety level of microwave radiation for children," Barrie says.[86] In other words, no safety level has ever been officially established for children, because there *is* no safe level. Children have weaker immune systems than adults, as they are not fully developed; their skulls are thinner; they are smaller and therefore absorb more radiation than adults; and they are being exposed at a much younger age and for longer than adults have so far been. Barrie has witnessed heart-breaking evidence of this, and he receives up to 1,000 communiqués a week from people all over the world, seeking his help and advice. He also regularly receives calls from concerned parents and many others trying to deal with the harmful effects of microwave radiation from WiFi and other sources. The following excerpts from just two of those telephone conversations (with mothers in the UK)[87] reveal the true and heart-breaking extent of the harm.

"My daughter has just died. I am holding her hand. She has just had her 11th birthday and she was number 11 to die since the transmitter for WiFi was put near her and others' desks."

"My child is one of several with cancer/birth genetic problems. These only started after the transmitter was turned on. My worries are two-fold and take every second of my life. Will my child ever marry or find a partner and be happy? What will happen when I die? I know I will die worrying. Regardless of who is to blame, it is me, the mother, who carries guilt and responsibility."

Barrie has no doubts about the extreme harm caused by WiFi, and he feels very strongly about it: "Anyone who puts WiFi into a school should be locked up for the rest of their life," he says. "They're not fit to walk on the surface of this planet, because they haven't looked at the research and, whatever incentive they have, it's not worth the genetic problems that parents are going to face with their children when they're born."

These genetic problems result in a lifetime of agony, worry and guilt, not just for those parents, but also for generations to come, since the genetic deformities will get handed down and will affect the women's ability to reproduce later in life.[88] "Children are both neurologically and physiologically different from adults," says Barrie. "A child's brain tissue and bone marrow have different electrical conductivity properties than adults', due to their higher water content" …which means that children can absorb 10 times more microwave radiation than adults. Permanent low-level microwave exposure can induce chronic nitrosative and oxidative stress, damaging the cellular mitochondria, Barrie explains. This stress can cause irreversible mitochondrial DNA damage, which means that any damage (genetic or otherwise) can be transmitted to all successive generations through the maternal line.[89]

Referencing university researchers, government scientists and international scientific advisors, Barrie reports that "a minimum of 57.7% of schoolgirls exposed to low-level microwave radiation (WiFi) are at risk of suffering stillbirth, foetal abnormalities or genetically damaged children, when they give birth".

Given the devastating impact of this radiation, parents have a responsibility to ensure that their children are not exposed to WiFi radiation at school …or at home. That is not to say that the mothers quoted above are to blame for what happened. They were not aware of the dangers—because governments failed to tell them and, instead, sanctioned the use of this dangerous technology. For those mothers who may have unwittingly exposed their children to harm, it's like being sent to prison for a crime they didn't commit, while the real perpetrators—the source of the harm and those who hide the truth—go free. And this is essentially what is happening.

Jenny Fry: 3 October 1999–11 June 2015*

To find your child hanging from a tree was not something I ever expected to experience as a mother. It is the worst nightmare imaginable, and one that I live with every day. I will never forgive those who allowed the use of this lethal technology [WiFi] to destroy my daughter's life, my family's life and the lives of other families affected by the unconscionable lack of safety and protection of children in schools. I will not rest until justice is found for what I consider to be the murder of my daughter by state incompetence—a tragedy that is all the more devastating because it could have been prevented, had the authorities heeded my repeated warnings.

The school authorities refused to believe me when I warned them of the dangers of WiFi radiation and the problems they were causing Jenny. Because she was so severely affected, my daughter was treated as if she was suddenly a 'naughty' child, despite her school record of being a well-behaved, hardworking child, with above-average intelligence …until WiFi was installed in the school. At the same time, the school uniform changed, with the introduction of blazers with pockets, which led to pupils carrying their cell phones and iPods in their pockets instead of in their bags …which, in turn, exposed Jenny to even more radiation.

When the school installed industrial-strength WiFi, Jenny started having difficulty holding her pen or pencil, concentrating, thinking and writing, which led to problems with many teachers. I was asked if anything had changed, at the next parents' evening. I was initially unaware that the school had installed WiFi, and it was only when the school introduced a policy of most homework being set online that I realized what was happening. When Jenny started having nosebleeds, we became aware of the health dangers of children exposed to WiFi, cordless phones etc.

Jenny tried so hard to do well and maintain her standard of work. When she became overwhelmed by the radiation and needed to leave the classroom, she would find another room where she could work. However, this led to detentions when teachers refused to believe that she was being affected by the WiFi, which also caused urine urgency, which resulted in more detentions and in teachers refusing to let her go the toilet, which created a lot of confusion and stress for everyone.

As a result of all this, her tutor gave up on her and no longer showed up at meetings. Incredibly, this tutor had told a couple of boys that they should go hang themselves and she would provide the rope. Is this what planted the idea in Jenny's head? Many children complained about this but were ignored. We also found that Jenny had written a paragraph in her English book, stating that it was against her human rights to not be allowed to go to the toilet. What torture for a teenager. Did the teachers expect her to wet herself in front of the class?

When exposed to WiFi, Jenny's symptoms included headaches, stress, nosebleeds, sleep problems, urine urgency, temperature control issues, fatigue, anxiety, ear noises and pressure, exhaustion, restlessness, confusion, skin rashes and irritation, joint pains, racing heart, hormone and cycle problems and difficulty concentrating and finding the right words.

As a dental nurse, I knew that cell phone use was associated with brain tumours and parotid tumours, and that cancer clusters have happened around cell phone masts. It was only when Jenny became ill that I became aware of the hazards of WiFi and cordless phones, and I was not aware of the related suicide risk until after her death. I also discovered that there was a hidden phone mast behind a tree on a concrete water tower, which had 4G switched on the Sunday before her death. If I had known then what I know now, my daughter and possibly two other pupils might still be alive.

My advice to parents would be to home-school your child if the school authorities refuse to switch off WiFi, or to set up your own education groups and schools. I am not against technology, which I find amazing, but WiFi technology is decimating our children's health. We must avoid irradiating children and go back to safe, wired Ethernet connections. Take a precautionary approach and inform yourself of the dangers.[90]

I will leave you with Jenny's words:

I have no hope for humanity. We are destroying this beautiful Earth and I'm not good enough with words to stand out from the crowd and somehow help humanity. I'm insignificant. I'm an insignificant number on someone's screen, and so is my whole life—just a tiny blip in the existence of the universe. I find it hard to be hopeful when I can barely enjoy anything anymore.

I have just returned form putting daffodils and tulips on her grave.

Contributed by Debra Fry, Jenny's mother, in January 2018.

Once we know the truth, however, we become responsible. Industry has a responsibility not to harm us. Governments have a responsibility to protect and serve us. And every human being has a responsibility to not knowingly harm anyone else.

Can you see the irony?

You love your children. You feed them healthy food, teach them solid values, make sure they get into the best schools, and do all you can to ensure their success in life …and then you unwittingly expose them to dangerous microwave radiation, every day of their young lives, greatly increasing their chances of serious illness, cognitive impairment, genetic damage, infertility issues and aggressive behaviour, not to mention social dysfunction and disastrous personal relationships.

What a tragic waste of your tender loving care and precious resources …and of life itself, in the wondrous untapped potential of children everywhere.

To grown-up children everywhere: this is the story of your e-life*

This is the story of your e-life, from the moment of birth. After the initial fanfare of your arrival, you find yourself competing for attention with a gadget. It photographs you and shares you with the world—you, this miraculous creation—and it is hard to get a look-in when it is always in your face. And that buzzing feeling through all your tiny organs... well, it's not good news. You're going to have to fight for your life from now on, with more toxins and radiation coming at you than tiny bods have ever had to endure ...and with far less of the love you need in order to deal with it all. You may get some moments of undivided attention, but as soon as you do anything—smile, grab hold of something, say your first word, walk your first step—out comes the Gadget, wedged between you and the love source, to capture it all so others can be impressed by what you've done. The Gadget takes precedence over everything. It may watch over you, but not like a dog or other living creature that would actually love you—even though it, too, will be largely neglected, in favour of the Gadget.

It's a lonely world you've entered, and I'm not sure what to say to reassure you. Even though you were born to bring love into your family, your most fundamental default setting has already been suppressed. As your little body grows, your heart will struggle and your spirit may go into hiding unless things change.

Survival instincts will kick in, because they must. And you may become temperamental, agitated, unsettled and cranky. You will keep reaching for love, beating the air with your tiny fists, desperate for attention, for that connection you so fleetingly felt, but the Gadget will almost always come between you. You will not know how to handle this and you will cry, have tantrums or retreat deep inside. You will long to feel safe, to be held and enfolded in love, without that thing intervening.

You will not know how to get through, but you will soon have your own Gadget, which you will use to distract yourself and numb the pain. You will try to find the love you lost and you will stimulate your little body with bright lights and games, feeling some life stir inside ...but never enough and never that same precious feeling you once felt. Your Gadget will never make you happy, but it's all you've got that you can really count on. It is always there and always on, and it will become your world. More of you has been suppressed than you will ever know, but you will keep trying to fill that gnawing emptiness, because that is what you were born to do—radiate love and spread it all around you.

If you are reading this now, remember that you were human once—and can be once again. Cut the wireless umbilical that has been leaching your life force. Ditch the vampire Gadget and come back to love and real life. Uncover your tender heart and entrust it to those who can relate. Break free from the artificial intelligence that will never bring you freedom. Strip away the layers of superficial solace and come home. Your love may be deeply buried, but it is there and everyone wants it. You belong in the real world of hugs and loving touch, not in some emotional vacuum that sucks in any hope of salvation. You have been there and you know what it feels like to be e-loved and empty-hearted. Be brave now and dare to stand alone in this sea of septic devices. The tide is turning. You can usher in the new wave of human connectedness and spiritual enlightenment that will finally make sense of your existence. Many are still lost and lonely. We need you to lead the way back to our hearts.

For those born in the early 1990s and later.

39 Testing our convictions

Every July in Horsefly, there is a musical festival—Arts on the Fly. Lewis has volunteered to help out, and it's interesting to see him approaching it with a fresh perspective. He is relatively unknown in this small community, yet he is quickly making his mark. In the process, though, he's becoming aware of how his former roles in business have shaped and compromised him. When we take on a particular role, we must then play within its limits, which means we limit ourselves—unless our role is that of disruptive thinker, tasked with changing and questioning everything. (I like that one.) If that were our own personal goal, we'd be far more expansive in our thoughts and actions, breaking through those confining limits and inspiring others to do the same.

So, I ask him, who will you choose to be in this community where nobody knows you? How will you choose to show up, what image will you project, and what story will you tell?

This reminds me that I must tell a different story about who I am. I must completely rewrite my story of EMF-induced harm, instead affirming that wireless radiation bounces right off me, like raindrops off an umbrella. I'm absolutely safe, no matter where I go or what I do. I thrive in any environment. The world is my playground, full of possibilities and opportunities that nourish, strengthen and support me in being fully me.

Given my fascination with human dynamics and figuring out how things work, inside and out, it feels wrong for me to be in this situation. How can I acquire so much wisdom and knowledge, yet be in a position of such weakness? I almost feel ashamed to not be physically embodying what I've been teaching for so long. *How can I know this stuff yet not be living it?* Yet, I have lived it, in the past, and I know how things work, but isn't that all the more reason for me to have somehow risen above this and not become a victim? It might seem arrogant to say that I'm too powerful to be affected by all this stuff, but isn't that true of us all? We all have the same physical, spiritual, neurological, emotional and mental faculties, which means that we all have the potential to be masterful human beings. Despite my moments of feeling as if I've failed to be powerful, I also know that we are only ever pushed down so that we can become stronger in fighting our way back up, building exceptionally strong emotional and spiritual 'muscles' along the way. This is how I now choose to see my current situation so that I can climb back up to—and beyond—where I was before.

But... back to Lewis. "If you were to reinvent yourself, what would you say?" I ask him. "Do you go into the community and say that you feel blessed to be an artist, that you love it, that it's how you discover who you are, that it's always been easy for you to paint, that your work is hugely sought after, and that you are constantly inspired with new images? Why not own *that* story rather than the one about a struggling, starving artist?"

"Because it's not true," Lewis says.

"But you can *make* it true," I say. "It's not yet true for me that I'm unaffected by EMFs, yet I'm claiming and affirming that as my new reality—the one I'm envisioning and creating out there in the quantum field, where it already exists as a potential."

I'm reminding myself of what I need to do and keep doing. Partners are handy like that, acting as sounding boards for our growth. We can get lots of practice telling them what we most need to hear. "The deeper truth is that I'm greater than my environment, greater than time and greater than my body, right? So I must be ahead of my time and step into a reality, in my mind, that has not yet taken shape in physical form. I must make it true in the moment of saying it. I must wear it, like a new coat I'm trying on.

"I want to hear your new story. Hit me with it. Give it to me with lots of colour, feeling and passion—your ideal reality now."

"I'm incredibly grateful for everything we have, everything we are and everything we have achieved. I'm loving our life—the beach, nature, our house and the artistic, creative lifestyle we're living. I'm deeply fulfilled as an artist, constantly challenging myself with new ideas and edgy concepts, and always going deeper into the process of discovery, with a beginner's mind. My work sells faster than I can produce it and I feel immensely gratified every time a painting finds a loving home. I have arrived. I have finally found my natural niche and the kind of peace that comes from doing exactly what I was born to do."

"I've never heard you say that before—that you're grateful for having a life that you love, right now," I tell Lewis. "I could actually feel you change as you said those words. Your whole demeanour changed, your energy lifted and your face lit up."

I don't think Lewis has any idea how powerful he is when he aligns with the deeper part of himself that wants to be expressed. (Yes, I know; it's true for me, too ...and everyone reading this.) It's not just about giving himself permission to finally *go* for it and be a full-time devoted artist. It's about *loving* his art so much that it fills him up and expands his vision of himself, his sense of self and his capacity for endless manifestation. It creates that *elevated emotion* that Dispenza says is so critical to creating the reality we want, out there in the quantum field. When we feel intensely positive emotions, it changes our energy field, which changes our reality.

"I could feel the power of you stepping into that future vision of yourself and your art," I say. "That alone could change how you paint from now on, if you can hold onto that feeling of excitement and gratitude for what's to come."

The power comes from feeding our ideal future reality as if it's current. Somewhere out there in the universe, in the quantum field, it already exists—whether it's a healthy, safe environment or just some better lifestyle that we envision. We just need to pull it to us and make it manifest in physical form. And it's only when we connect with that quantum realm that our brain takes the appropriate action and releases the chemicals to heal us or connect us with the outcome we seek. Time is irrelevant. The switch from despair to excited connectedness and being in the flow can be instantaneous.

**When we feel intensely positive emotions,
it changes our energy field, which changes our reality.**

We've both had our duels with despair and hopelessness, and we know how much effort it can seem to take to pull ourselves out of that state.

"If we can't switch into that mindset of it happening now, how else are we going to manage it?" says Lewis. "There's no logic to this stuff. We can't know what the outcome will be, just because we do certain things. We can only trust that the outcome will be positive, if we stay focused on that being our reality."

"I think the only reason we ever sink into despair is the belief that we can't have the future we dream of," I say. "If we absolutely knew that we could have it, we'd be so excited we'd hardly be able to contain ourselves. And we'd also probably value every minute we have here, knowing that we were going to be moving on and would never have this kind of experience again."

"So, here's an interesting question," says Lewis, and I can tell that he's about to challenge me. "Given where you are now, in the process of trying to become strong enough to withstand EMFs, consider this: If, tomorrow, someone offered us a beautiful home in Costa Rica, on the beach, and all you had to do was get on a plane and go there, what would you do?"

"I'd get on that plane," I say, instantly. "I'd find a way. I'd take a shielding net with me and I'd—"

"But would you need a net?" Lewis asks.

"Maybe not," I say. "If I was excited enough, I might not need anything, as long as I was prepared."

"But why would you need to prepare? Aren't you just getting back into the old logic of cause and effect if you react that way and prepare to protect yourself from harm?"

"Yes, darn it. You're right. I am. I'm still thinking that way. I need to own that strength now and start living that way, rather than allowing my fear of being harmed to determine how I behave."

This is the challenge—embracing a future reality now, even though my mind is objecting furiously. If I let go of the vision and the excitement of going to our own place in the tropics, I feel terror at the very idea of getting on a long-haul flight with no escape from the high levels of radiation that might make the trip unbearable—even deadly.

"But your fear comes from believing that that radiation will harm you further," says Lewis.

It's true. Fear primes the body for an assault, putting all systems on red alert and sending a powerful signal of vulnerability, which is the opposite of what needs to happen for the brain to re-wire itself as being strong, invulnerable and resilient, and for the body to respond to that new strength and counter whatever is happening on the outside.

Our excitement about life and our faith in ourselves being powerful, masterful beings must outweigh the fears we have about not being in charge of our lives.

40 A vision of the future

We're having a lazy late breakfast, looking out at the trees, blue sky and the bright-red umbrella on our deck.

"Has Manuel fixed the boat?" Lewis asks. "I want to get out on the water today and take some photos of the pelicans as they're diving."

"I think so," I say. "I saw him working on it earlier."

"Great. I'm really looking forward to doing some abstracts based on pelicans—something that really captures their spirit."

"Can't wait to see those," I say, as I ponder my day. I think I'll go for a swim. It's a perfect day for it—warm sunshine, hardly any wind, yet not too hot for some sunbathing on the beach afterwards.

"This afternoon, I thought we could go into the village," Lewis is saying as he munches noisily on his Ryvita crackers, loaded with peanut butter and apricot jam. "We could have a coffee at that little café we went to last week, with Rosie and Michel. They might be there again today."

"Perfect," I say. "I'm going to have one of their yummy chocolate cookies."

"It's so fantastic that we can do this again," Lewis says, beaming at me. "Just to be able to go to a café together, after all this time, and not have it affect you."

"Doesn't touch me!" I declare, referring to the WiFi at the café—and the cell phones still carried by some people in the village, although far fewer than before, due to the greater general awareness. I am proud of myself. Here I am engaging in life like a quasi-normal person. It feels good—not just for me but also for Lewis, who has had to do so much on his own while I was recovering.

I'm feeling strong and healthy, my body tanned, toned and relaxed from sunbathing, swimming and long walks on the beach. In white cotton shorts, navy T-shirt and purple flip-flops, I'm finally living the life we've always envisaged. All the cranial inflammation and nerve-zapping has gone and my head is once again peaceful—apart from all the creative ideas zooming around, which I welcome as a natural part of being engaged in life and loving it.

"I still can't believe I've got my hearing back!" I say. "Can you believe it, Lewis, after all this time?"

"It's the best news I've heard in the last 15 years," Lewis says, "since you said *I do*."

"I get so excited sometimes I can hardly contain myself," I say, jigging up and down on my seat. "I think you're going to have to keep me on a short bungee cord so I don't go into orbit."

"I want to celebrate every minute of every day," says Lewis, "but then I'd never get any painting done—although that's a kind of celebration in itself, I suppose."

"Yes, definitely. I can't think of anything that makes me happier than seeing you painting and loving it."

"Shall we take the Aston Martin to the village?" Lewis's new canary-yellow convertible is his favourite possession and he jumps at any opportunity to take it for a spin.

"I thought we could go on the bikes as it's such a lovely day," I say, but he knows I'm only teasing him. It's also the perfect day for driving with the top down, our hair blowing in the wind as we soak up the sun, salty smells and scenery around us.

"I must remember to water the herb garden before we go," Lewis says.

"Maybe Silvia could do that. She'll be cooking Rendang curry this evening, don't forget." Rendang curry is my favourite meal of all time—a typical Malaysian dish made from a rich blend of aromatic spices and meat stewed slowly for hours until it's falling-off-the-bone tender.

"And don't forget that your agent is dropping by tomorrow," I remind him. "How many paintings is he taking with him this time?"

"Ten, I think. I have more, but some of them aren't quite dry yet."

"Wasn't there a guy in the village who wanted to buy some?"

"Yes—that architect who lives in the villa up on the hill. He wants four of my earlier ones, I think."

I can hardly believe how perfect, easy and rewarding our life has become. To have gone from being severely restricted, socially isolated and functionally impaired, to being mobile, active, socially engaged and creatively fulfilled is like a dream come true.

It is the dream we are cultivating, as we sit here having breakfast in Horsefly, pre-living our future ideal life in the sun, as if it were already happening. Somewhere, out there in the quantum field, it already is.

41 Maligned and misaligned: a delicate balancing act

How many negative thoughts do you have in a day, or even in an hour? How you treat yourself plays a pivotal role in your health and in what you attract into your life. Repeated thoughts and beliefs cause neurons to fire and wire together, building a strong, healthy body or a vulnerable unwell one, depending on the quality of your thinking. Your brain is in charge of that, and you are in charge of your brain. Keeping your thoughts, words and actions coherent, positive and in alignment with each other therefore has a powerful impact on your personal reality.

Many of us have strong values about life and the way we live it. We may like to think of ourselves as having integrity in the way we do business, for example. But having integrity means being at one with ourselves. In other words, having our actions in alignment with our thoughts, words and values. Yet how often are they? How often do we feel one thing but do another? We say we respect the environment yet we keep buying plastic containers or bags. We say we want to be healthy, yet we malign and mistreat ourselves in lots of ways.

Being out of alignment in our behaviour has a significant impact on our lives. It means that we are at odds with our internal guidance system and we therefore transmit mixed messages about who and what we are, which usually results in mixed results in business, relationships and other interactions. Being physically misaligned is also significant, and one usually promotes the other.

Finding our balance

I know what it's like to be off kilter—not just because I experienced dizziness due to EMFS and the tumour, but because brain surgery knocked my skull out of alignment. It was several years before I realized that this was affecting me, causing blockages in my neck and a build-up of tension in my head. If circulation of nutrients is impeded and if communication between the body and the brain is restricted, it's impossible to be healthy, or even comfortable in your body. This was one of many factors that needed to be addressed for me to regain my balance and well-being ...and for me to be more resilient against EMFs.

Most of us are out of physical alignment, and it is rare to see beautifully upright, correct posture. But the issue goes much deeper than that. According to Pete Egoscue, an anatomical physiologist who developed a revolutionary non-invasive system for eliminating chronic pain,[91] the body is very precisely structured to allow for the flow of high-wavelength energy down through the spine to nourish the entire system. When we are out of alignment, this life-giving energy cannot flow as it should and the body is compromised on many levels. Joints and muscles are affected, as is our emotional state.

If you think of how most people spend most of their day—either looking down at a cell phone in their hands or at a computer screen—it's not hard to see why so many of us are out of alignment. Factor in stress, poor posture, anxiety (which affects breathing, which affects muscles), and it's easy to see why the body might have difficulty holding or returning to its optimal position.

Fear is another crucial factor in our ability to remain healthy. "[...] fear can be a disease—a killer, the mother of all lethal infections—because it diverts energy away from healthy physiological processes," says Egoscue, in his book, *Pain Free Living*. "Organs can be drained of important resources and left terribly vulnerable." This is particularly relevant for those affected by electromagnetic radiation, since the fear of being harmed further depletes the body's resilience. Fear is particularly dangerous, Egoscue says, because it locks you out of the present moment and blocks the awareness you need in order to be in touch with your body. Fear creates physical, emotional and psychological stress for the body, clouding our vision of what's possible, while numbing us to its damaging impact.

Although Egoscue does not directly address the issue of harmful radiation in our environment, he explains how misalignment of the musculoskeletal system profoundly affects our resistance to illness or whatever else comes at us.

The primary purpose of the musculoskeletal system is, he says, to download and circulate high-wavelength energy to fuel the sixty trillion cells in the typical adult body. This puts an entirely new spin on our everyday functionality, and understanding this crucial factor can help us regain strength and resilience.

"When you plug into the universal power grid by balancing your posture and drawing on its high-wavelength energy," Egoscue says, "the mental and physical static quiets down; in its place are clarity and focus. The incoming energy flow smooths turbulence by augmenting and supporting the metabolic power required to renew the body's cells." We need a steady flow of healthy energy to fuel, repair and operate the body's many systems. This energy also facilitates the removal of wastes, fights disease and enables us to be more connected to the feelings that accurately convey to the body what it needs in order to function optimally.

This life-giving energy plays a key role in keeping us healthy and in countering stressors and toxins. Having a strong, properly aligned and engaged physical body also helps to orchestrate the countless chemical, electrical, biomechanical and cellular processes that take place throughout our lives. We are like antennas, conducting energy from above and below, and tuning in to what is happening inside and all around us. Vital communication takes place via the spine and our nervous system, constantly alerting the brain to the adjustments or recalibrations it needs to make to keep us in balance.

**Having a strong, properly aligned body
helps to orchestrate the countless processes
that take place in our bodies throughout our lives.**

Physical misalignment is a reliable indicator of the body's inability to take on energy supplies, Egoscue says. A misaligned body triggers a host of warnings that activate hormonal responses that affect your mood, respiration, blood pressure, energy levels, and resistance to illness. This misalignment can inhibit circulation, pinch nerves, starve muscles and prevent a smooth flow of oxygen, information and energy throughout the body. When this happens, we begin to deteriorate, since the body cannot function as intended and toxins can build up in the tissues. The body can get locked into a state of tension or rigidity and we may instinctively compensate for the parts that no longer move very well. "Stiffness and immobility are two characteristics of a corpse," says Egoscue, and fluid movement is therefore essential to good health.

When we understand how much our thoughts and feelings affect our physicality, we realize that a flexible mind cultivates a flexible body—and vice versa. Maintaining a healthy balance in our thinking enables us to start dissolving the stories about ourselves that create tension and keep us stuck—physically as well as emotionally.

How our stories take shape

The stories that evolve out of our early programming shape our personalities and our physical bodies, consolidating what we've been led to believe is the truth. We all create stories in our lives, yet they often prevent us from healing, even if we consciously seem to be doing all we can to get well. We create these stories, Egoscue says, because we are afraid to go inward to obtain and marshal the resources needed to recover or sustain our own health. Our stories are designed to shield us from fear so that we can go on living in the presence of it. But numbing ourselves to fear or anxiety also causes other parts of us to shut down, disconnecting us from our feelings and our sense of ownership for our reality.

Our stories define and shape us to such an extent that Egoscue has been able to identify certain personality types with particular physical and functional characteristics. He describes the fact-collector, the pessimist and the cynic, for example, all of whom have their own distinctive areas of pain, tension, rigidity and emotional characteristics that affect their musculoskeletal system and, therefore, their ability to be well. Simple exercises targeting each type enable individuals to regain their flexibility, structural integrity and healthy flow of energy. Instead of deepening the story about how tough it is to heal the body (resorting to invasive surgery, taking drugs, or curtailing activities because of pain or inflexibility), individuals can re-align their bodies, eliminate pain, regain their vitality and, in the process, defuse some of their limiting beliefs about what's possible.

We can use our stories to keep ourselves stuck and to justify being unwell—*it's hereditary, I've always been like this, doctors say nothing can be done etc*—or we can start to understand that we embody many of the stories we have, allowing them to physically limit and define us.

While correcting physical and emotional misalignment may not seem directly relevant to addressing the effects of EMFs, it is clear that it affects our strength, balance and resilience, keeping our bodies dynamic and ensuring a healthy flow of life-enhancing energy.

42 Making a conscious commitment

It is a gentle day for late September, puffs of warm air buffeting my skin but not insisting. As I cross the grass to the cabin, I see a moose down by the water, and I pause to observe its majestic passing. There are dragonflies everywhere, their neon-blue bodies criss-crossing the air like mini-drones on an important reconnaissance mission. A large yellow insect circles overhead, its wings clapping like a pair of castanets, applauding the skies. The chipmunks, too, are active—popping up from their hiding places to bask in the warm sunshine, then scuttling out of sight as I approach. Yellow garter snakes make an occasional sly appearance from under the cabin steps, their vividly striped bodies a brilliant splash of colour against the bleached wood.

In this peaceful setting, it seems inherently wrong to be worried—about anything. But I'm aware of a deep gnawing fear inside, fuelled by increasing cranial inflammation, hearing loss and balance issues. *What if there's another tumour on the other side?* This is my fear. *What if I lose my hearing altogether?* This seems almost as terrifying as dying and is, in a sense, a form of death. It would mean the loss of so many precious things—hearing the sound of Lewis's voice, being able to engage in conversations, enjoying the sounds of the natural world around me, music, laughter, waves on a beach, and my ability to stay safe. I cannot imagine not being able to hear anything, although I'm getting a taste of what that might be like. Yet there are many things that I could never have imagined happening. The fact that our world is intentionally being bombarded with microwave radiation is madness enough, and I still wake up some mornings thinking it must all be a bad dream. This cannot be happening. No leaders in their right minds would support this kind of thing.

Yet we are all leaders in our own lives, many of us being pushed to push back. For me, it's *do or die*. I'm aware of the healing that needs to happen, but I don't feel I'm fully engaging in it. I know the theory, but my heart is still away on holiday somewhere, refusing to come home to deal with things. Since heart and soul took off on that package deal before my surgery, I haven't heard a peep from either of them. Not that I can blame them. I want to get away from me, too.

After doing all I can to heal myself on my own, I decide to get some outside help and support. And I know exactly who I want to work with …if she's willing to embark on this journey with me. Lucy Sanford has already done this work, healing herself from EHS and becoming a certified Electromagnetic Radiation Specialist (EMRS) along the way. She embodies what I believe to be vital components for healing: a spiritual approach, an understanding of the deeper drivers of disease, a highly analytical mind (I've finally met my match), an understanding of the principles of quantum physics and neuroplasticity, extensive knowledge and personal awareness of the effects of EMFs, and a commitment to not engage in the negative stories, patterns or memories that keep us stuck.

Healing can be a rocky road—not because healing is necessarily difficult but because it can be hard to let go of old patterns. With the right beliefs, self-talk and actions, healing can be easy and fast, and there are countless stories of spontaneous healing occurring in all kinds of situations. Given the nature of our minds, however, and our deeply entrenched subconscious programming, the resistance to positive change can be huge. You may experience moments of euphoria when you make a breakthrough, discover some deeper truth or start an exciting creative project that you feel will take you towards the life and the health that you seek.

When you understand and start tapping into universal intelligence, everything feels possible—and it is. But the old perceived reality can come crashing back, testing your conviction in your faith to create positive change. Your symptoms may worsen or you may wake up feeling depressed and hopeless, convinced that you will never be able to heal yourself. But this is just a reflection of how stubbornly the mind wants to hold on to the old ways of thinking and behaving. Being aware of this resistance is not always enough to break free of it, however, and it can be hard to catch yourself at your own game. Having a healing 'buddy' or mentor to help keep you on track can make all the difference.

I first connected with Lucy when I was compiling material for my WHO document, and I included part of her personal story in the report. I sensed a kindred spirit and a shared conviction that electromagnetic sensitivity was far more than just a physical reaction to our irradiated environment.

I asked Lucy if she felt angry about all the harm caused to her by the radiation, as so many other electro-sensitive people do.

"After more than 20 years of feeling unwell, I think I was more relieved than anything else to finally have an answer and to know what was wrong," she said. "I was frustrated at not being able to do things or to go into restaurants, but my focus was on getting to a place where I felt safe and getting well, so I was never really angry."

Lucy preferred not to mix with people who resented their condition and felt like victims of what was coming at them. "To get better, I had to stay away from those negative feelings," she said. "I had to not go there myself and not be around people who were angry. Those emotions were very disruptive to me and I could not have healed if I'd stayed in that emotional environment."

I think about this dichotomy in my own life. Even as I'm doing all I can to heal myself—eating well, exercising, taking supplements, feeding my ideal future reality, meditating—I may be simultaneously cancelling it out with fearful or negative thoughts, old ways of doing things, or concerns about the future. Being in alignment with my purpose (to heal body and mind) requires that all of me be onboard with the program. Anything less than congruity sends mixed messages—not just to my brain and body, but also to the quantum field where things coalesce before materializing in my physical reality.

Yet Lucy is aware of what's going on and is disturbed by the emerging realities, such as the roll-out of 5G, with no clear vision of how they can be addressed. What she *has* managed to change is her own reaction to all the man-made radiation. She can now tolerate it, although she chooses not to live in it and has created a healthy, low-EMF environment in her home. But she can go into restaurants and cafés, take flights, and be close to people using a cell phone, without feeling any effects.

I think of Dr Erica Mallery-Blythe and other EHS specialists and scientists who have confirmed the impact of EMFs on the blood (using live-blood-cell analysis), even in those who don't feel the radiation and are not aware of being affected by it. I ask Lucy if she thinks she's still being affected by the radiation, even if she doesn't feel it.

"I agree that we're all affected, in some way, but I'm no longer getting symptoms," she says. "I know it's there and that it's dangerous, and I choose not to live in it. When I first started doing the work to get well, I thought I had to also change my view of electromagnetic radiation being bad for me. But I still think it is bad for us, even though I've managed to get my body and mind strong enough to not react to it."

Lucy did, however, become hypersensitive again, after getting three CT scans. Not realizing until after the fact that these scans emitted over 1,000 times as much radiation as a normal X-ray, it took her a while to figure out why she was once again getting symptoms. Once she realized what had happened, she was able to eliminate her symptoms and once again regain her health by working with the brain's neuroplasticity and applying the principles of quantum physics to change her personal reality.

Now that I've become so aware of all the electromagnetic radiation around us, it's hard to imagine why anyone would knowingly subject their bodies to this kind of non-stop assault. A densely populated, high-EMF environment also emits a very different vibe, and the level of meaningful connection between individuals is greatly reduced or fragmented, due to the always-on, constantly stimulated and distracted nature of those glued to their wireless devices. Privacy, personal boundaries and respect for others all seem to go out the window when a cell phone beckons, pulling the recipient out of the present moment and away from any ongoing in-person human interaction.

Perhaps it does all come down to frequency. If we raise our own frequencies enough, can we remain unaffected, even as the radiation levels continue to rise? Even if we do, though, what about plants, animals, insects and the environment itself? No matter how much we might manage to change or individually master ourselves, the ongoing radiation emissions still affect all forms of life. But that can change, too, if enough of us return to our spiritual selves and start living our lives from that perspective.

"Being involved with like-minded spiritual people is what really saved me," says Lucy. "That's what nourishes me and gives me vitality."

Yet, even in those circles, there seems to be a lack of awareness of what's going on. "Why aren't they talking about it?" Lucy wonders. "Surely we can't just allow this abuse of our planet to continue if we are committed to living a spiritual life."

Lucy wants to raise awareness in a non-judgemental way so that people understand the consequences of what we're all doing. "It's very hard for me to watch these things going on and not raise awareness about it," she says. "I'm sometimes asked to do a presentation, but I don't want to instil fear. I think people are already too exhausted and discouraged about our environment, so they turn off. They don't want to hear about it."

Lucy feels that the best we can do with the current technology is change the way we use our devices, such as cell phones, while creating healthy sanctuaries in our homes so we can get restorative rest and give our bodies a break from the radiation. Then, when we're out in the world, we can deal with it all much better.

I like to envision a safe, innovative technology that provides all of the convenience and benefits without any of the downsides. Given what's possible when we apply the laws of quantum physics and envision living in a wonderfully healthy environment, it's perfectly feasible. If we collectively feed a positive vision of vibrant good health in a healthy environment, it will happen.

People are already doing something about this, Lucy tells me, with thousands of people around the world doing meditations to heal the Earth. "But," she laughs, "most people are tuning in to these meditations on their cell phones!"

Dr Joe Dispenza, for example, created a global meditation—Project Coherence: Raising the Earth's Electromagnetic Field—in which over 6,000 people from 77 countries have participated.[92] As he says on his site, research has shown that when we cultivate the emotional states of caring, love and compassion, our hearts expand and we radiate coherent energy that can be used to benefit both ourselves and the world. The more satellites of people around the world are broadcasting a coherent organized signature, the greater the influence on the unified field around the Earth as well as on every individual. When two or more waves oscillate in tandem and are vibrating at the same frequency, we experience a phenomenon known as *constructive interference*—the two waves come together and create a resultant waveform with much greater power and amplitude. Similarly, when people share a common purpose and focus together on a specific goal, their combined intent creates coherence in the quantum field.

In working with Lucy, I realized that some deeply entrenched subconscious patterns around being unwell were preventing me from bouncing back. I needed to address the underlying issues so that I could build greater strength and resilience.

It's not that any of us consciously want to be sick, of course (although there can be some unconscious perceived benefits, such as avoiding something we don't want to do). But trauma, loss or unmet emotional needs in childhood can result in real physical issues, which can then become a pattern, creating a cycle of ill-health that can only be broken with conscious, loving awareness. We all create very clever strategies and ways of dealing with emotional challenges and/or physical threats, setting the scene for a lifetime of distorted perceptions and heightened reactivity to certain triggers. It doesn't really matter whether the trigger is real or perceived; it's our reaction to it that reinforces particular patterns and expands the neural networks that then cause our situation to also expand. Unless we understand this process and break those cycles, our lives can become self-fulfilling prophecies.

What we think and feel has a huge impact on our lives, and out there, in the quantum field.

"The unconscious parts of the ego will use real-life situations to keep you stuck and keep you sick—if that's your particular addiction," Lucy says.

I know that, even though our ego strives to keep us safe, it often misinterprets its job description, protecting us from things that we ideally need to address and resolve in healthy ways, instead of running away from or reacting to them. Because the body gets addicted to the chemicals generated by certain repeated emotions, it will create a need for those chemicals to continue being produced—in the same way that people become addicted to their wireless devices, which produce the feel-good neurotransmitter dopamine.[93] (See Chapter 37 for more on addiction.)

For those who are unwell, whether it's due to EHS or something else, this means that symptoms will continue to manifest, providing seemingly valid evidence of the external environment being the cause of their condition. (This is not to say that harmful EMFs in our environment are not an issue; they certainly are, but we can address them on more than the physical level.)

We tend to use external circumstances to confirm our pre-conceived notions of how life works, yet our circumstances are a reflection of what is going on inside. Subconscious limiting beliefs can be difficult to root out and they can seriously cramp our style without us realizing what's going on. We inevitably encounter resistance when we try to change those old beliefs, and it takes discipline and a strong desire for positive change to break through.

All the cells of our body have their own intelligence, and they are constantly being re-programmed by our beliefs and emotional investments. Unless we consciously change those beliefs and break free of emotional dependencies, our cells will want to consistently feel the way they do whenever we encounter illness, helplessness, negativity or limitation. This is just as true for those who are electro-sensitive, since exposure to radiation can emotionally trigger us in many of the same ways that we're triggered by an abusive partner, an angry boss or any other person who violates our boundaries or adversely affects us in some way.

This explains why we tend to attract partners who feed our patterns, triggering us in ways that enable us to keep having the same reaction, while feeding the neural networks that influence our reality. It's not much fun when this happens, and we tend to blame our partner, our bad luck with men/women, or the general lack of suitable partners, unaware of our tremendous power to attract what feeds our addictions.

**The degree to which we blame others
is the degree to which we feel powerless over our own lives.**

We must remember that we are electromagnetic beings, with thoughts that produce an electrical field and emotions that generate their own magnetism. So what we think and feel has a huge impact on our lives—and out there, in the quantum field. While the harmful EMFs in our environment may be very real and a growing threat to all forms of life on Earth, feeding that belief does not serve us in our quest for a healthier life and body, and for global solutions.

Working with Lucy is helping me to stay focused on the bigger picture and to not get sucked back into the drama or fear of being harmed by a hostile environment. I must stay connected to the deeper truth and my innate capacity to change my personal reality. Even though I'm familiar with many of the universal principles we're working with, I still find myself forgetting what I most need to remember. The ego is a very slippery customer and our subconscious programs are extremely stubborn, hanging on for dear life for as long as they can. We therefore need to become objective observers of what's going on inside and out, so that we are no longer caught up in the drama or reactivity of our programing and can clearly see what's happening.

This reminds me of two crucial components of healing or recovery from any kind of trauma or dysfunction: healthy, enlightened support and a meaningful human connection. We may have wonderful friends to whom we turn in times of stress or loss. But the truest friend is the one who reminds us of our greatness, supports us in being all that we can be, never lets us get caught up in drama, negativity or self-flagellation, and keeps us on track with the deeper truth that's always trying to emerge.

My goal is to re-wire my brain so that my body and mind believe me to be safe, healthy and resilient, no matter what. In my joyous future reality, my heart (versus old negative patterns) is running the show, I am centred and present (no longer reacting to old triggers), I travel with confidence and engage with others (no longer fearful of exposure to WiFi or other EMFs), and I have absolute faith in myself and in universal intelligence to handle whatever challenges I encounter, while retaining and boosting my health.

The rapidly advancing threat of global 5G makes it clear that we must 'power up' as fast as we possibly can, using our minds, our hearts and our higher capacities to feed a vision of a healthy environment. While it is devastating to learn of the impending harm that will inevitably result from this invasive new technology, we must remind ourselves that we are being pushed to re-connect with our humanity and to do the very opposite of what 5G and the Internet of Things (IoT) represent. As quantum observers and creators, within a rapidly growing community of many millions worldwide, we can have an impact far beyond what our logical minds believe is possible.

"The goal is to harmonize our energy; identify and dislodge the unconscious energetic patterns that keep us stuck in dis-ease; step out of fear; find balance and coherence in chaos; transform our ego so it works for us rather than against us; and become the superheroes we are meant to be."

—Lucy Sanford

43 Update from the wilderness

It is our last week on the off-grid property and I wonder if it has been worth it. After the EMF issues with the solar power and satellite Internet, the stress of encroaching wildfires, being virtually alone on this isolated property, and not having easy access to healthcare or amenities, what have I gained? How much have I healed and learned? Did I do what I had hoped to do by coming here?

These are not easy questions to answer, since I've learned things I didn't expect to learn. Yet, in other respects, I haven't made the progress I'd hoped to make. In a way, it feels as if the healing process has barely begun. Separating myself from the crazy wireless world has definitely been beneficial. I'm more relaxed, more at peace within myself and more connected to nature. I've slowed down and my mind and body are less agitated. I'm sleeping better and I feel calmer when I eat. But these are all things that I do on my own, without any human interaction and without being affected by cell phones, WiFi or other potential triggers—including people. Removing triggers is not the same as healing. Yet some physical healing has occurred, thanks to the peace and serenity of this place and the lack of usual everyday events and demands, such as social outings, appointments and work.

I'm also much more aware of my own patterns and how I deal with stressors. Despite the relative peace of this place, we have nonetheless had our challenges: dealing with the unexpected EMFs here, preparing for a possible evacuation away from the forest fires, and grappling with our own inner demons. This is where most of the work has taken place—inside ourselves. Being together 24/7 in an isolated environment inevitably triggers our own stuff, bringing it to the surface so we can address it. In many ways, we've done that very well, stepping back from the issue and seeing it for what it is. Sometimes, though, we've been sucked back into the drama of things, all our fears and frustrations feeding the charge. *Where do we go from here? What's next? Where will we live? What can we do?* The need to control our future can feel very real if we forget who's really driving the bus. Yet our need to *know* what's going to happen next can keep us stuck in old patterns, since the familiar and the known are based on memories and past experiences. Only by embracing the unknown do we allow new experiences and nice surprises to come to us. Although clinging to the known might seem safer, the unknown holds the gems of our untold greatness.

With just a week to go before our lease on this place expires, we still have not found another place to live. For the past month, Lewis has been scouting around for a rental and he's becoming increasingly agitated as I've rejected every place he's found. It's almost the end of September and winter will soon be here. But none of the places feels right, and not just because of EMF issues. Yet I'm not worried, and this, in itself, is huge progress. To not be worrying about finding a safe place, away from the dreaded wireless technologies and the electrical grid, is a very positive shift. Fear just makes things worse, and I'm determined to never again let it overwhelm me, as it has done in the past. Instead, I'm trusting that we will find the perfect place ...and we do.

If someone had said to me that we would be offered the use of a beautiful home, free of charge for the next seven months, and that we wouldn't even have to pay for firewood or utilities, I might have been just a teeny weeny bit skeptical (even though such things are possible, of course). I might have asked *how* this would come about and who on Earth would give us such a huge gift, in this tiny community where so few people know us. But I know it's not our job to figure out the *how* of things. All we need to do is focus on what we want and trust that the universe will deliver.

With just a few days to go before our lease expires, we find ourselves moving to a beautiful large property, just 3km from Horsefly, off a paved road, with all the amenities we could wish for and more. Despite the fact that there's a smart meter about 20 metres from the house and an Internet satellite dish outside the master bedroom, I know it's the right place for us—not just because it feels right but because I'd asked for a sign. Weeks before we moved, I said to Lewis that the perfect place would have a table-tennis table. None of the other places we'd looked at had one. Yet, here, tucked away at the back of the huge workshop beside the house, is a brand-new table-tennis table, just waiting for us to use it.

When we replace the existing cordless phones with corded ones, switch off the WiFi in favour of a wired connection, shield the smart meter with aluminium mesh, and turn off all the breakers we don't need (such as the ones for the microwave, some lights/electrical sockets, the washing machine and other appliances that we only use occasionally), the levels of microwave radiation go right down. The electrical levels, however, remain higher then we'd ideally like, for optimal health, even when the entire electrical panel is switched off. Only then do I realize that there is a transformer about 10 metres from the house, instead of being out on the road, as they usually are. Clearly, this is what's raising the EMFs inside the house.

Despite my initial dismay at this discovery, I realize that it's there for a reason—and not just to regulate the voltage coming into the house. I know that I must embrace these challenges in order to build resilience and emotional/spiritual 'muscle', rather than trying to have everything perfect so that no evolution is required. I get it. This whole place is a gift, exactly as it is. Whatever challenges I perceive to exist are there to make me stronger. They provide the resistance I need to work with in order to grow. They offer the perfect opportunity for me to see what's possible when I apply the principles of quantum physics I've been studying. I can become stronger than my environment and stronger than my body, transforming the old pattern of reacting with fear, trepidation and defensiveness to any apparent threat.

Even though the electrical fields in our bedroom are relatively high, periodically going into the orange zone on my electrosmog meter, I choose not to see them as a threat to my health. Instead, I declare that my entire body and the immediate area around it is a 'green zone', emitting a strong, healthy aura that ensures resilience, cellular regeneration and ongoing rejuvenation. I see it as being stronger than whatever EMFs might be coming at me from the outside, and I catch myself if my mind tries to pull me back into the old way of thinking. *Stop, stop, change! I am a green zone, I am a green zone... I am stronger than my environment and stronger than my mind.*

Relaxing into this new mode of positive projection feels like a huge relief and a huge shift from my previous state of ongoing anxiety, which was all too readily fuelled by external circumstances. This state of empowered acceptance also generates its own kind of magic, cultivating the flow of universal intelligence and all it has to offer. Just two days after I chose not to allow the high electrical fields from the transformer to be an issue, some BC Hydro contractors show up at our door. Apparently, the pole on which the transformer sits is due to be replaced ...which offers the perfect opportunity for the transformer to be moved further away from the house. Not a big deal and it won't cost you anything, the contractors tell me, and I marvel at how beautifully things flow when I get out of the way.

Making a conscious shift from being a victim to a creator is the most powerful thing we can do to take back control of our health and our lives, whatever the circumstances. When we realize that we are part of an infinite field of universal consciousness, intelligence and pure potentiality, we realize that we don't need to struggle to make things happen; we don't need to worry; and we don't need to get caught up in the dramas of life. We can tap into that field of potentiality to create what we want. We can ask for help and let it go, trusting that it will come back to us in some perfect scenario that we could not have orchestrated with our logical minds.

When you make this shift, Dr Deepak Chopra says, "You realize that the world is a mirror of your thoughts, your feelings, your desires, your interpretations. You know that every situation, every relationship, every event you experience is mirroring something inside you. [...] If something you're experiencing in your life is causing you to be unhappy, you recognize that it's your creation. Otherwise, you stay in victim mode: *Poor me. This is happening to me, and I am powerless to change it.* Why wait for the world to change when, in fact, you are creating the world? Whatever is happening is because you are creating it, so you ask yourself: *What do I need to shift inside of me so this doesn't happen?*"

While it may be difficult to accept that we have created the harmful EMFs in our environment, we have all contributed to this situation. Due to our uninformed choices, our lack of awareness of the dangers (and our failure to do our own research/due diligence), and/or our passive acceptance of how things are (all of which are driven by the deeper subconscious programs within us), we are very much the drivers of our own destiny, whether we are consciously aware of this or not.

Moving from victimhood to creatorship is a profoundly spiritual shift that changes everything. It expands our perception of what's possible. It transforms the way we relate to self and others. It motivates us to nourish and care for our bodies. It prompts us to live with discernment and make conscious choices. It generates a healthy hunger for awareness, inner peace, spirituality and happiness. And it inspires us to utilize our physical reality as a springboard to greatness.

44 I hear you, body; I hear you, world

With my concerns about progressive hearing loss in my left ear (with my right ear already deaf due to the surgery), I realize that I've given more thought, energy and feeling to the probability of losing my hearing than to the possibility of regaining it. To turn this around, I must fully apply the principles of neural reprogramming and quantum physics, while bearing in mind the law of attraction. What we focus on is what we get, so focusing on loss or harm promotes exactly what I don't want.

I must shift my focus, envision having perfect hearing, and feel the excitement and gratitude of once again hearing perfectly in both ears right now. I must also mentally conjure up images of me living a rich and joyous life with perfect hearing, as well as generating the positive, uplifting emotions that I would feel in that reality.

For every day for a month, I'm spending time doing that—and exclaiming at every opportunity (such as when someone tells me something), *I hear you!*

I think back to our month in Granja, where all the barking dogs kept me awake at night. I did everything I could to block out the noise—used earplugs and expletives, sealed the windows, pleaded with the dog-owning neighbours—and that is when the hearing loss began. Some people suggest that hearing loss is the body's way of getting you to listen to your own wisdom, which you may be forced to do if you can no longer hear—or maybe don't want to hear—what anyone else is saying. (Hey, I hear you!)

Before Granja, I experienced years of fragmented sleep due to the snoring of a certain partner. Since sleep is one of those non-negotiable necessities of life, no one should have to go without it. I made some unhealthy compromises, however, and it took me a while to address this issue. In the meantime, my body was getting a very clear message every night that I didn't want to hear what I was hearing. Healthy boundaries must be proactively created with our words and actions, instead of the body bearing the brunt of our unhealthy compromises and shutting down whatever parts of us we seem to be disowning.

Figuring out our internal dynamics, our subconscious programs, and the ego's clever strategies for trying to keep us 'safe' requires a lot of self-examination, honesty and discipline. We may prefer to avoid exploring what's buried beneath our everyday awareness. But if we're ill, in pain or being harmed by our environment, we need to rally all our healing forces and ensure that all of the self—conscious and subconscious—is committed to us getting well.

Can I do this? Of course I can. But will I? Will I stay committed to the challenge every day, will I refuse to entertain even one second of doubt, and will I catch myself in the act of anticipating further harm? Or will I pre-live that life of perfect hearing and spend time in a state of blissful gratitude for having regained that fabulous faculty?

Either way, you'll be hearing from me.

45 Being the change we want to see

It's the week before Christmas and I have a raging toothache. After trying for months to find a dentist who understands the dangers of EMR and is willing to accommodate me, I've arranged to see one in the nearest large town, an hour away, even though they have WiFi and were unwilling to turn it off when Lewis asked about this a few months ago. This time, I decide to call and take a different approach. I chat with a young receptionist, who is very friendly and loves my Irish accent. I ask about the various dentists at the clinic, to see which one might be the best fit for me. Then I mention needing to be as far away from the WiFi as possible, as I'm sensitive to the radiation. She is interested to know more and we chat for a few minutes about this. She has no awareness of the health effects, but she's open to hearing me. She then suggests I come in to see how things feel and books me in with the dentist furthest away from the WiFi router ...assuming that I'm able to handle the EMFs when I come in. I feel a warm welcome, with the promise that I'll be taken care of.

This is a very different conversation to those I've had with other dentists, and it feels good to consciously take a more receptive approach and have it lead to a more positive outcome. Before, I would have been frustrated that no one understood the dangers and was unwilling to protect my health ...and my defensiveness was no doubt apparent in the way I spoke. Now I know better. I know that, since I'm in charge of me (creating my own scenarios, through my projections and beliefs), I'm giving myself the opportunity to practise what I've been learning and to show myself just how strong and resilient I can be. No more being a victim. Now, every challenge is an opportunity to see what I'm capable of.

The levels of microwave radiation at the clinic are not as high as expected, and I decide that I can—and will—deal with them. I could have done this sooner, had I changed my attitude sooner, but that's okay. No more making myself wrong, either, since that's just more of the negative programming that so cramps our style. I remind myself, too, that I must be the change I want to see. If I want to be treated with respect and consideration, I must express those qualities in all my interactions.

However, when I return for an exam to see what work needs to be done, I discover that the levels of microwave radiation are over 100 times higher than when I first checked. I find this alarming, even though I know it is another opportunity to practise being stronger than my environment and not have it affect me.

Despite my best efforts, however, I feel depleted by the exposure and I am not looking forward to going back for treatment.

After reflecting on this during the week before my next appointment, I call the clinic again and speak to Michelle—the young female dentist who examined me. I explain my concerns and ask if the WiFi can be turned off during my treatment, given the very high levels of radiation and the fact that the computers at the clinic are all hardwired, so WiFi is not even required by the staff in order for them to operate.

Unlike many of my previous exchanges with health professionals, I remain very calm and open to being heard and helped, saying that I understand her situation. I also say that I wish I'd listened to others who, in the past, had told me what I was now telling her about the dangers. If I had done so, I might have avoided getting a brain tumour. So you understand, I say to Michelle, why I take this issue very seriously and do what I can to protect my health.

She did and she responded positively, changing my appointment to her lunch hour and …unplugging the WiFi router. When we originally asked for this to be done, prior to seeing the dentist, we met with resistance. Having established a rapport, however, we achieved the desired outcome. Having that connection changed everything, and the conversation ended on a very warm, friendly note. My treatment a week later was (dare I say it) almost enjoyable, with both Michelle and her assistant being every bit as gentle and caring as I could have wished for.

Given what I've learned about the positive impact of an emotional connection, I know that my treatment with this dentist ended up being far more restorative and less harmful than it might otherwise have been, thanks to her compassion and willingness to accommodate me. I was able to get the work done without being exposed to harmful radiation, while relating to her on a much more heartfelt level. We all know how much better it feels to be treated by a doctor who cares and listens to our concerns than by one who doesn't.

My experience was a reminder not just of the importance of changing my attitude in order to generate a more positive outcome, but also of the need to appeal to the humanity of those with whom I wish to connect in a meaningful way. We all want to have loving, caring connections in our lives. If they are missing in our exchanges, it is up to us to cultivate them.

46 Troglodytes, unite!

I used to own a Noddy car. Unless you're from Ireland or the UK, you probably won't know what this is , and I'm sorry if you missed out on this wonderful aspect of childhood. Noddy is a character created by Enid Blyton, a bestselling author of children's books from the 1930s until she died in 1968. Noddy had a very funky yellow car, with chrome bumpers, bright-red wheel arches and a big fat horn. So did I, when I was only 3 years old. Mine was a pedal car, but I could work up quite a speed, racing up and down the cement path that bordered our garden. I could reverse and parallel-park by the time I was 4, and I had to show my Mum how to reverse out of the driveway when she was learning to drive in her 30s.

I still miss that car and wouldn't mind having an adult-sized pedal-powered version now. Although I'm not about to go and live in a cave, I do love low-tech stuff and I appreciate the craftsmanship that goes into making something so solid, functional and enduring (not to mention quirky). If I still had that car now, it would be a collector's item. I remember the trauma of having it taken away from me when my Mum gave it to the 'junk' man. (There's gratitude for you, after me teaching her to drive!) When I lost that car, I lost a special piece of my childhood identity. I had no time for dolls or any of that girlie stuff; cars, bikes and anything mechanical held far more fascination for me than tea parties or getting dressed up.

Using our hands and our bodies is what we're designed for.

I still feel that way, and being electro-sensitive has only fed my fondness for things I can operate without electricity. Using our hands and our bodies is what we're designed for, and I will always choose manually operated devices over electric or electronic ones …and eco-friendly over toxic. No GPS for me. I prefer to look at a nice big map to find my way around, and to do my sums (at least up to double digits) in my head or on paper, rather than using a calculator. Both are good for the brain, keeping it agile and working both hemispheres. In the kitchen, we use a very chic manual coffee-bean grinder, a manual mincer for making burgers, and a classic 'plunger' cafétière for making coffee—all wonderfully free of EMFs and transferable overseas, since no voltage is involved. We also have solar-powered desk lamps and, if we move to a warmer climate, I'll be buying a sun oven.

My most recent low-tech, low-EMF purchase is an AlphaSmart word processor. This is basically a keyboard with a very small screen that displays about five lines of text at a time. It runs on three small batteries, which last for almost a year, and it emits almost no EMFs. It's ideal for electro-sensitive individuals or for writers who don't need to be online or don't want the distraction of e-mails or texts coming at them. It includes a spell-checker, eight separate document folders and a word-count function. It's simple, very low-tech and won't crash on you. I can take it anywhere and will never have to plug it in. When I've finished whatever I'm writing, I can safely transfer the content to my laptop and save or send from there.

But such items are becoming harder to find as the demand for increasingly sophisticated wireless electronic devices continues to grow. It's up to us to create a demand for the good 'old-fashioned' stuff so that it doesn't disappear forever (like my Noddy car). The AlphaSmart is no longer being made, as far as I know, but various models can still be purchased online.

Here in Horsefly, there is little demand for high-tech gadgets, with the emphasis being more on solid machinery and self-sufficiency. Most people build their own home; many grow their own food and create some kind of cottage industry; and some even make their own musical instruments. (The number of talented musicians and artists here rivals that of any major city, but without all the high-tech trappings. Perhaps that's no coincidence.)

The homes are beautiful structures, built with eco-friendly materials, creative designs and almost no 'smart' stuff. Some operate off the grid but most have smart meters, the installation of which encountered little resistance from residents, due to a general lack of awareness of the dangers. Most people in Horsefly are against the installation of cell towers here. Yet many homes have cordless phones—again, simply due to a lack of awareness of how the devices work. Most people also have satellite Internet, since there is no facility for telephone- or cable-based broadband Internet connections. Despite the otherwise healthy lifestyle, there seems to be a significant incidence of cancer, which could be due to (or exacerbated by) the high levels of radiation from the cordless phones and satellite dishes (as well as in-home WiFi, in most cases), in combination with other lifestyle/dietary factors.

With a little more knowledge and awareness, however, combined with the existing skills and appreciation for living in and off the natural environment, small communities such as this have the potential to be electromagnetically healthy places to live. When we combine an understanding of nature and of our electromagnetic bodies, with an understanding of the science that explains the interrelationship between the two, we can find creative ways to be high-tech *and* healthy. There are many wonderful innovative eco-friendly products and technologies out there, on the sidelines, just waiting for the demand for them to increase.

As an added bonus, the people of Horsefly bring new meaning to the term *community*, demonstrating more kindness, generosity and eco-friendly wisdom than anywhere else we've lived.

Sounds like a no-brainer, in terms of where we should settle. On the other hand, it's winter for half the year and the mosquitoes can be ferocious in June. Nor does it fit our vision of living by the sea in a warmer climate—which means I can't walk on the beach or wear my flip-flops (except indoors). You may not think that such things are important, but flip-flops are very good for the sole. And they're not just some cheap foot flap. They enable your feet to move the way they're meant to, boosting circulation, working your musculoskeletal system and helping to keep things properly aligned. Our feet are not meant to be imprisoned in unbending boots, growing pale and pudgy from lack of movement and sunshine. Flip-flops provide a great workout for your legs, which are attached to your hips, which support your torso and organs… you get the idea.

Healing requires a return to wholeness, which means looking at the body holistically. Addressing the various parts of the whole will never lead to a complete solution. In the same way that allopathic medicine tends to target specific parts of the body as if they were independent (usually failing in its attempts to restore wellness), trying to resolve the EMF issue without resolving all the other de-natured aspects of our existence will not take us to a place of balance, well-being or fulfillment. It's also important to be happy, which comes from being in the right place with the right mental and emotional attitude.

If we stick around in Horsefly long enough to help build greater awareness (and there are already some significant movers and shakers here who have succeeded in keeping WiFi out of the local school, among other things), and if enough eco-conscious individuals support the natural lifestyle, this little place could well turn out to be a model for low-EMF living. If that happens, and if I get really good at this quantum physics stuff, I might be able to improve the climate or even get the Pacific Ocean to come to me. Of course, that might mean that Vancouverites living on the fourth floor of their apartment block would have to take a boat to work, and the people living in the floors below would have to get their homes converted into submarines. There are easier ways for us to manifest what we desire, without having to go to such extremes. I remind myself to keep things simple, to not let my mind take over and start Worry War III, and to trust in the universe to keep bringing us nice surprises, while we keep feeding our vision of a healthy life in the sun.

There can be resistance to change, even in small communities such as Horsefly, and that's understandable. People move here for a reason—to get away from the rat race, to be their own boss, to buy their own land, build their own home, be in charge of their own lives—and they don't need any outsiders coming in and telling them what to do.

A small town or village that's struggling and looking for new blood, creative ideas and ways of injecting some new life into the community may be a more open, receptive environment for something new to come in. Plus, if enough electro-sensitive people were interested in becoming part of such a community, they could end up being the majority, which would make things a lot easier in terms of the kind of eco-friendly, low-EMF culture they might wish to create, while benefitting everyone.

It's much more exciting and compelling to create something new than to try to change an existing situation.

In the same way that some hitherto unknown town has become a centre for something unique, based on an innovative idea, some small communities could end up being magnets for innovation and progressive thinking. Think of Bilbao, in Spain, which was a failing industrial city that had become rundown and had nothing to look forward to …until they came up with the very bold idea of building the Guggenheim Museum. Famous architect Frank Gehry was commissioned to design it and it cost $68 million to build—and another $35 million for the art that was displayed inside. Within five years, however, they had made $168 million out of it and it had stimulated all kinds of businesses, putting Bilbao on the art map and making it the envy of the art world.

It's much more exciting and compelling to create something new than to try to change an existing situation. Imagine a town dedicated to innovative eco-friendly technologies, personal empowerment, art and creativity, and a culture of collaboration for the benefit of all. Think of the businesses and cottage industries that could be set up, the opportunities for training and educating other communities wishing to adopt the same model, the holistic centres that could offer all kinds of alternative therapies, and the benefits of being part of a like-minded community dedicated to excellence, exploring new dimensions, and seeking new ways to protect the Earth and tap into our co-creative powers. It could be a hotbed of creativity, becoming a magnet for others wishing to be part of a cohesive, open-minded, values-driven, holistic approach to life.

For eco-conscious, electro-sensitive bods seeking a healthy place to live, it pays to get creative and to think beyond the usual reactive survival strategies (living in a cave, retreating to the wilderness, barricading yourself behind miles of shielding foil and wire mesh). Many small towns and villages in Italy are looking for ways to revitalize their economies, and the mayor of one Italian town launched a campaign in 2016 to attract more residents, offering them low rent and a €2,000 cash incentive if they moved there. This offer has since been rescinded,[94] with the Mayor begging people to stop calling him after thousands tried to take him up on his offer. The overwhelming response is very good news, however, since it shows how willing people are to move to a remote location and how much demand there is for creative initiatives like this. There are also some eco-villages in Canada,[95] and other small towns, such as some of those in Saskatchewan, that have the potential to become low-EMF communities.

It would mean getting the mayor or municipality to commit to not installing any cell towers or other EMR-transmitting technologies nearby, and to supporting the low-EMF concept. Apart from those who are electro-sensitive, many others would welcome an escape from the world of technology, and a holiday in a EMF-free zone would hold many attractions, while providing economic benefits for the whole community.

When young people leave for better jobs and more excitement in the city, such communities often experience a loss of purpose and vitality, with few resources or options for sustaining their existence. With the right approach, these towns and villages could become healthy, economically viable communities for those with electro-sensitivity, becoming centres of excellence in eco-friendly living and innovative technology that provide huge benefits without any unhealthy downsides.

These dying villages are both a reflection of the unhealthy shift towards a technologically driven lifestyle and an opportunity for creative individuals to bring them back to life with a focus on eco-friendly housing, organic farming, cottage industries, healthy telecommunication technologies and a true sense of community through collaboration.

We don't need to become cave-dwellers in order to distance ourselves from the assault of man-made radiation. Creating a simpler way of life, in tune with nature and our own natural rhythms, while tapping into the same degree of creativity and innovation that has led to so many technological advances, offers the potential for us to create exciting, healthy, sustainable lifestyles.

47 Reality check: who's really in charge?

I talk to many people affected by EMR who are trying to get the government to change things, and most of them tell me that the healthcare authorities are the problem. If they could just convince the authorities of the evidence and get them to see the need for stricter guidelines and more stringent safety levels, things would be okay. *Then* things would start to change.

But the problem is not just the healthcare authorities, the governments or even the offending wireless telecommunications industry (although they have seriously harmed a significant percentage of the population). The problem is the people. We've been programmed to defer to authority, to be passive, to have things done for us, to not fight back, to do whatever it takes to survive. We have opted out of being responsible for our own lives, choosing convenience and ease over confrontation or everyday activism. We want doctors to give us a pill to make us better. We expect politicians to fix homelessness, poverty, high taxes, crime etc. We expect service-providers to have researched all the latest technologies and to make things safe so that we can indulge in the latest gadgets and get on with living the good life in the fast lane. We expect farmers to keep growing our food and delivering it to supermarkets. We expect to get free WiFi, free software, free online services, free e-books and so many other things that we now take completely for granted. We may have more freedom, more technological expertise and more abundance than ever before, but we are more profoundly disempowered and disconnected from the truth than at any other time in our history. We have abdicated control over our own lives in all the ways that count.

**We may not want industry to be running the show,
but we have all bought a ticket to watch it.**

Things are the way they are because of the way we are. Our governments are the product of our lack of responsibility for our own lives. As a result, almost every aspect of society has, it seems, been hijacked in the name of progress, convenience, jobs and technological advancement. Health, food, waste management, politics, industry and the environment itself—all have been commandeered by government authorities and those with a vested interest in making us dependent on their products and services.

Yet this should not surprise us, since we gave away responsibility for these things many years ago. Most importantly, we gave away responsibility for our selves, which resulted in our need for others to fix us, feed us, govern us, psycho-analyse us, acknowledge us, like us, protect us, go to war for us, and generally provide for our every need without us having to do much at all. We can take drugs to make our symptoms go away; we can pluck all our food right off supermarket shelves without having to worry about crop failures or bad weather; we flush the toilet and our waste is swept away to some unknown place—out of sight, out of mind; we put our mountains of plastic into recycling bins and keep on buying; and we trust that governments are taking care of our environment, while we ourselves take almost no responsibility for our everyday choices or their impact.

But, Olga, I care about the environment. I recycle, and that's good …right? Recycling requires using even more resources to process things so we can use them again. It's not going to save our planet and, in any case, we're recycling the wrong stuff. Recycling glass is a good thing. But recycling our limited beliefs and negative emotions should not be allowed. It's very bad for the environment.

We are being irradiated beyond our control and without our permission because we have already given our tacit consent. We have never fought back. We have not done our own due diligence as the technologies were being rolled out. We have not taken responsibility for our own safety, health or awareness. Most of us (including me) have never stood our ground on political or social issues, instead expecting others to do the work and be the activists that we all need to be in our own lives. And every one of us, at some point and to some degree, has said yes to what's happening. We might know better now, especially if we have been harmed by all the radiation, but the prevailing ignorance is just a continuation of what has gone on for far too long.

Recycling our limited beliefs and negative emotions is very bad for the environment.

Awareness of this massive violation of our rights and decimation of our health can be seen as a push towards empowerment—the biggest, strongest push we've ever had. But if you don't strive to reclaim your autonomy, you're out of the game. You can't score any points or win the last round. Your voice won't be heard. You won't be accountable to yourself. You become a victim rather than the victor you're meant to be. You've missed the whole point of the resistance being presented to you so that you fight back with equal strength and reclaim your right to exist and thrive.

This is not happening *to* us but *for* us. It might seem as if we're being targeted or victimized, but what's happening to us is the product of our dysfunction—the inevitable outcome of generations of subservience, low self-worth, deference to authority, fear of not being good enough, wanting people to fix us, dodging confrontation, surrendering our autonomy, and not taking responsibility for our own lives. And that dysfunction, which is the root of all that ails us in our world, is caused by the negative programs that get downloaded into our subconscious minds by default and without our awareness.

Through religion, schooling, politics and our upbringing, we are programmed to see ourselves as powerless to change things, and we're rarely taught that we have the right, the responsibility and the capacity to be powerful. We unthinkingly accept what's done to us without realizing that it's designed to give us the opportunity to push back so that we develop strength and emotional 'muscle' in those very aspects of self that were made wobbly by our early negative programming.

The deeper truth is that we are more powerful than we can imagine. We are not victims and our lives are not random. Every weakness we develop in our early years has its counterpart in our evolution. If we were abused, we attract more abusers until we push back and reclaim our autonomy and self-respect. If we feel insecure, we attract controlling or domineering partners whose behaviour challenges us to be strong. We are being pushed by every aspect of our dysfunctional lives to step into our power and to start being the autonomous, majestic creators we are designed to be. Representing the ultimate wake-up call (as graphically demonstrated by the widespread harm we've caused to our planet), the progressive incapacitation resulting from the electromagnetic radiation in our environment may well bring us to our knees before we get the message.

Let's face it...

The rapid, ongoing degeneration of our bodies and our planet is unsustainable and will very soon threaten our survival. We cannot go on like this. You don't need to be a mathematician, a physicist, an ecologist or a bee-keeper to know that critical eco-systems are out of balance, populations are exploding, resources are dwindling, people are getting sicker, new epidemics are raging across the globe, industry is running the show, natural resources are being poisoned, communities are breaking down, debts are spiralling, economies are failing, the incidence of suicide and depression is rocketing, our food is de-natured, healthcare is all about pharmaceuticals, our children are being drugged up to the eyeballs, the elderly are being sedated into oblivion, our atmosphere is polluted, our food supply is threatened, marine life is dying, our oceans are clogged with plastic, and the enormity of it all leaves us in a state of perpetual mind-numbing denial and paralysis.

*Yet we have all the resources and solutions we need to address this crisis ...*if we shift from a position of subservience to one of autonomy. We have the means to thrive while enjoying life to the full and protecting our environmentally based life-support systems in the process. What we have yet to realize, as a species, is that we can thrive in ways beyond our imagining when we work *with* our natural resources rather than exploiting them. Never before have there been so many eco-friendly technologies, clean-energy options and innovative products at our disposal. More and more creative people are doing amazing things for our planet, and they are driven by a desire for eco-excellence, rather than a need to compete for profit.

If we were all driven by that same quest for excellence—in ourselves and in all that we do—we would be truly astounded at our capacity to create a world of harmony, peace and creativity.

48 Perception is everything

What's your story about EMFs? Whatever it is, it will tell a much bigger story about you and your life. We all have stories about how life works, how unfair things might be, and how deserving, important or lovable we are. Yet all of these stories are like movies being projected through the lens of our subconscious onto the screen that we call life. They don't reflect reality; they reflect our *perception* of it.

And perception, as biologist Dr Bruce Lipton tells us, is everything. The author of *The Biology of Belief*, Dr Lipton has provided biological evidence of the key role played by our perceptions in influencing our reality. He shows how perception even has the power to change our genes,[96] thereby eliminating the widely held belief that our genes are part of our destiny and therefore cannot be changed.

Having the right mindset and perception of life is crucial to having the life that you want.[97] With a victim mindset, even a supposedly EHS-friendly place can turn out to be a problem, as it did for me. Yet, with the right mindset, a place with a smart meter, satellite Internet and a transformer nearby turned out to be perfect, and a gift that was freely given, with very little effort required by me to make it happen.

This seems to defy logic, yet it makes perfect sense when you remember that logic is just the result of mental constructs that produce what we have learned to expect them to produce. Our higher mind and universal intelligence can do far more impressive things than merely confirm our pre-programmed beliefs.

I challenge you to challenge yourself—to call yourself on your own stuff, your perceived limitations, your resistance, your denial and whatever objections or justifications you come up with to convince yourself that you can't have what you want (which keeps you stuck in being a victim).

It's not just about healing our bodies or leading a healthier lifestyle. It's about activating parts of us that may never have been activated before. It's about graduating to a whole new level of human functionality and spiritual supremacy that enables us to go far beyond our old ways of perceiving and transforming our reality.

Since science has shown that, by changing our perception, we can change our genes, we can also change our destiny. If there's a history of cancer in your family, do you want to sustain that belief and to perceive your own body as being the inevitable victim of that genetic inheritance? Would you consider getting your breasts removed if breast cancer 'ran in your family'? If you knew that you could re-program your genes by changing your perception of how things work, would you not want to change your mind about that? And if genes can be modified as a result of our perception, is it not likely that those original 'cancer' genes were the result of someone else's limited perception?

There are so many big questions that emerge when we contemplate letting go of deeply held beliefs and convictions. Why would we not want to change our genetic destiny if we had the power to do so? Why are so many of us subconsciously addicted to being sick? Why are we addicted to suffering when we have the power to live a life of ease, heartfelt connectivity and joyous fulfillment?

Many of these questions are equally valid in the context of EMFs. Why do we choose to live in a world of dysfunction when we have the ability—and the responsibility—to set ourselves free? Of course, many of us may not know that we have that ability, and we all reach that awareness in our own good time. But, once we know it, we often still refuse to accept it, even if it means that we experience discomfort, dysfunction and disease, as a result. Yet there is always some perceived payoff for such choices—not having to change, not having to take responsibility for something, or simply because our denial has become an unconscious habit.

Most of the challenges we face today are the result of our collective, complicit collusion with those in power.

If we don't want to change, we must accept the world as it is, as well as our part in making it the way it is. If we do want to change and to take responsibility for our current reality, we must give it everything we've got, because nothing less than total commitment to our conscious evolution will bring about the transformation that needs to occur inside and out.

In the same way that no one wins if the wireless industry continues to benefit from our disempowerment, we all benefit if even one of us becomes empowered. We can understand how this might be so when we understand that we are all part of a unified field of energy and therefore all interconnected. Quantum physicists discovered a strange property in the subatomic world called 'nonlocality', whereby quantum particles are connected and remain connected, continuing to influence each other, regardless of time or space. "There may be no such thing as place and no such thing as distance," says

George Musser.[98] "Physics experiments can bind the fate of two particles together so that they behave like a pair of magic coins. [...] They act in a coordinated way even though no force passes through the space between them." Those particles might zip off to opposite sides of the universe, he says, yet still act in unison. In doing so, they transcend space and our concept of locality.

> ## Our sense of the universe as an orderly expanse where events happen in absolute locations is an illusion.
>
> —George Musser

This ties in with the theory of morphic resonance, originally developed by British biologist Rupert Sheldrake. This followed on from his theory of formative causation, which states that the forms of self-organizing living things—everything from molecules, cells and organisms to societies and even galaxies—are shaped by morphogenetic fields (groups of cells able to respond to discrete, localized biochemical signals that define the biology of all living things, guiding the development of an organism as it grows, and causing cells to assume their intended function/nature). "The fields organizing the activity of the nervous system are likewise inherited through morphic resonance, conveying a collective, instinctive memory," Sheldrake says. Each individual both draws upon and contributes to the collective memory of the species.

Sheldrake believes that these fields differed from electromagnetic fields because they reverberated across generations with an inherent memory of the shape and form of cells/species. His theory resulted in a radically new interpretation of how memories are stored and how we inherit genetic material. "Memory need not be stored in material traces inside brains, which are more like TV receivers than video recorders," he says, "tuning into influences from the past." Our biological inheritance therefore does not need to be coded into our genes, since much of it depends on morphic resonance from previous members of the species. Thus, he says, we inherit a collective memory from past members of the species, while also contributing to the collective memory and affecting other members of the species in the future.

When we realize that we exist in a vast interconnected web of energy throughout space and time, we begin to see what's possible via that much more powerful 'worldwide web'. Through this web, which some call the quantum or unified field, we have access to the limitless possibilities that exist in the universe. As demonstrated by quantum physics, we have the capacity to 'collapse' those possibilities into our physical reality, using an elevated state of consciousness. Even the act of placing our attention on something can change it.

In applying those principles and in expanding our vision of what's possible, we can change our reality. While we may have originally been programmed to think and act a certain way, at an age when we had no say in the matter, we are now, as adults, free to change our minds. We no longer need to perpetuate an unhealthy co-dependence. With conscious awareness, we can break free, and many of us are becoming aware of our greater potential and learning how to tap into the quantum field of infinite possibilities. The more of us that do this, the faster the tide turns in our favour.

49 Electronic gadgets: mirrors of our misplaced mastery

Our biggest flaw as humans is our denial of the obvious. Our disregard for scientific evidence and for the fact that disease is consuming us faster than we can document it proves that our denial is still our most stupendous and uniquely human achievement.

Yet it's not that we are stupid; it's that we have suppressed and lost touch with our phenomenal wisdom, creativity and power.

Technology has evolved faster than we could ever have imagined, yet our emotional and spiritual evolution has lagged far behind. Our personal evolution has been so profoundly stunted by our dysfunction and so rapidly outstripped by technology that most of us are incapable of integrating these sophisticated technological developments into our lives in a balanced way, while respecting, staying connected to and being nourished by nature. Even though our bodies, hearts and spirits are screaming for our attention, we find more and more ways—and more and more technologies—to drown out the alarm bells and numb ourselves to our pain. And the sheer speed of technological progress prevents us from physically evolving fast enough to develop ways of protecting ourselves from microwave radiation.

We will do anything, it seems,
but give up the technology that is literally killing us.

Even so, our capacity to feel and sense emotions, telepathically know things, experience compassion and empathy, transcend pain, access higher planes of consciousness and heal our bodies is beyond the reach of even the most sophisticated computers.

All this shows us just how far, and in how many ways, we have strayed from who we really are. Almost every technology we have developed has its counterpart in our higher faculties. If we learned how to activate our supernatural powers, how to 'make things matter' by engaging with the quantum field, and how to master our minds and bodies, we could do many of the things that our electronic devices do for us today. That might not seem as exciting or as convenient as using a gadget, but there's nothing more exciting than creating magic in your life. Once we step into creatorship, we ease back from consumerism; we lose our fascination with external devices; and we start to experience the profound fulfillment that only comes from being who we're meant to be.

If we worked with the neuroplasticity of our vastly under-utilized brains, we could do many of the amazing things that our electronic gadgets do.

Despite our phenomenal brainpower, however, we have allowed ourselves to become increasingly mechanized. Yet our humanity is our most important quality and the key to our survival. Without it, we disconnect from each other and from our innate faculties, using apps, electronic gadgets and all kinds of high-tech devices to do the things that we used to do with our hands, heads and hearts. In the process, we lose our connection to our natural internal and external environments, along with the vital physical, emotional and spiritual nourishment that comes from being connected to both.

What we have achieved technologically, with all our electronic devices, is a direct reflection of what we are capable of achieving within, using our higher faculties. Our gadgets are an externalization of our power, making us powerful by proxy, which pales in comparison with being consciously powerful ourselves. Mirroring our misplaced mastery and dazzling us with their wizardry, our gadgets keep us focused on externalities and oblivious to our phenomenal internal powers.

Using our multi-media

Our bodies are the media through which we experience, process and generate life, and this is where we must focus if we want to change anything. They provide a home for our heart, a vehicle for our brain, and an anchor for our soul. Through these various media, we can create new neural networks that generate new realities and the kind of connectivity that can blow our minds. While the various forms of social media may feed our need for stimulation, engagement, inspiration, creativity and connection, the body's media are the true media of transformation—our media of expression and evolution.

Networks, media, connectivity: can you see the parallels? These are the ideal things for us to work with, but *inside*, not out there in some reality created by our limited beliefs. It is in the process of consciously transforming ourselves that we tap into the higher faculties that enable us to transform our environment.

50 The effects of electro-magnetic radiation: 10 lessons learned

1. What you don't feel can still be very real. This is the hardest thing for us to wrap our brains around. Electromagnetic radiation is invisible, odourless and (for most of us) intangible, so it's hard for us to see it as being harmful—even if, subconsciously, we might sense that it is. Since EMR affects us at the cellular level, we may only become aware of it being a problem when physical symptoms occur or a disease develops and forces us to take notice. How long that takes depends on our individual degree and duration of exposure, the amount of stress in our lives, and our physical resilience/overall health. **Remember: just because you don't feel it doesn't mean it's not affecting you.** Think of carbon monoxide, asbestos, lead and smooth-talking men in fast cars with lots of money. They can all creep up on you without you realizing it.

2. We're hard-wired for denial, although you might disagree. None of my (ex)friends use a microwave oven, knowing that it's harmful, yet they all use a cell phone, WiFi, and an iPad (all of which emit high levels of microwave radiation). Microwave radiation has been used by the military as a weapon since the 1950s, but it's not harmful when it's used for *non*-military purposes …right? We all love the convenience and the feeling of significance that come from being wirelessly connected 24/7, and we don't want to give it up. Denial is inevitable when there seems to be so much at stake, and we tell ourselves that it's safer, better for our business, and essential for our work to have this wireless access. And all those lovely funky gadgets are so much fun! How could such sophisticated technology be *harmful?* Even when I realized that this radiation was harming me, I still didn't protect myself until it was too late. My denial cost me dearly. If I could choose, retroactively, between giving up all wireless devices 100%, and avoiding brain surgery as well as retaining all of my wonderful hearing, youthfulness and flexibility, guess which one I'd choose.

3. You'll blame your symptoms on everything else. *I* did, for years, and I so regret not making the connection sooner. But I understand why I didn't, even though that's difficult to accept, in hindsight. *If you don't feel the effects,* *you won't care. If you don't care, you won't look. If you don't look, you won't see. If you don't see, you won't believe. But the evidence is there.* Of course, your insomnia, anxiety or hormonal issues could be due to something totally unrelated to electromagnetic radiation, but it may well be a factor. Because EMR affects the body at the cellular level, penetrating membranes, depleting the immune system, disrupting hormones, affecting fertility and crossing the all-important blood–brain barrier that's so essential to protecting the brain from toxic substances, it affects every single body system, organ, gland and function. Rather than leaving this till last, when trying to find the root cause of your condition, consider it up front, immediately and save yourself a great deal of pain, money and eggs (the ones inside you that can get wi-fried).

4. EMR makes everything worse. There's a code of honour about not hitting someone when they're down ...isn't there? Anyway, if your body has been weakened by ongoing exposure to harmful radiation, it starts to lose its resilience and it can't bounce back the way it used to. Whatever new stressor comes your way is going to hit you that much harder. Doctors who understand the dangers of EMR say that, even if you get a stroke that's caused by something else, the effects will be far worse—and a full recovery far less likely—if you've been chronically exposed to electromagnetic radiation. Whatever part of your body happens to be the weakest (due to other stressors in your life) becomes your Achilles' heel—the part that will collapse most readily and succumb to illness or disease. Exposure to high levels of microwave radiation can be the last straw for people who have managed to keep going, despite not feeling super-healthy, but have no reserves for dealing with additional stressors.

5. Everyone has their tipping point. The effects of electromagnetic radiation are cumulative. With ongoing exposure, they build up in your body. Therefore, the more you are exposed, the greater the impact on your body and the lower your tolerance. As the levels of radiation continue to increase all around us, with no sign (as of early 2018) of things slowing down or the authorities coming to their senses, your body is like a ticking time bomb. You might feel okay now (and I hope you continue to feel that way for a long time), but everyone has their tipping point of intolerance and our bodies are not equipped to deal with this kind of extreme, non-stop electrical interference. I've heard countless stories of people reaching their tipping point when some additional factor entered their lives—the installation of a wireless smart meter, the stress and grief of losing a loved one, getting a new iPad for Christmas, moving into a new Smart home, or getting a new job that required hours of cell phone use every day. Something, at some point, will inevitably tip you over the edge ...and you won't see it coming.

6. Most doctors/neurosurgeons are uninformed about EMR and may lead you further astray. When I had to undergo surgery for the removal of the acoustic neuroma caused by microwave radiation from WiFi/cell phones, I was exposed to high levels of that same radiation in the hospital where the surgery was performed. Afterwards, I was advised to get regular MRI scans to check that there had been no re-growth. Yet the MRI machine produces extremely high levels of the electromagnetic fields that I was trying to escape, and I subsequently heard stories of several people who *became* electro-sensitive as a direct result of having an MRI scan. Do your own due diligence. Don't blindly trust what doctors tell you, no matter how well-intentioned they might seem. Fear is a powerful tool often used in medicine to compel you to take the conventional/drug-based route. If a doctor or neurosurgeon tells you that there is no evidence that microwave radiation causes tumours/cancers (among other things), do not accept these unfounded claims; they are clearly uninformed and their ignorance could cost you dearly. (Medical students are not taught about electro-sensitivity in medical school.) Also bear in mind that admitting to this correlation and warning people to avoid exposure might well constitute a conflict of interest for someone whose livelihood depends on performing surgeries or treating you with drugs.

7. Technological terminology can be deceptive. Everyone loves WiFi and cell phones, don't they? What could possibly be harmful about something that opens up a whole new world of limitless connectivity and fun? If we call it what it really is, however, it doesn't sound quite so benign. Let's say you're getting poor cell-phone reception in your home, and you call up your service-provider to complain. What are you really asking for? *"You're not beaming enough microwave radiation into my home. It's only irradiating some of the rooms and some of my family members and pets but not all of them, and I want more—in my bedroom, my children's bedrooms and through every inch of my property. If you can't send me more radiation, at greater strength, I'm switching to another network. I need this radiation to be available throughout my house, penetrating every wall and every person in it so that I don't have the unbearable inconvenience of going for one second without it."* Is that really what you want?

8. Ignorance (of EMR) is anything but blissful. There are some huge ironies in the ignorance around electromagnetic radiation. Take, for example, the mother of the teenage boy who started getting epileptic fits and wants her son to have his cell phone on him at all times, so he can be in touch in an emergency. Or the elderly woman with worsening heart issues who insists on having her cell phone beside her in bed at night, in case she needs to call emergency services. Or anyone who has insomnia, anxiety or other physical/ mental health issues and uses their cell phone to research the condition online to try to help themselves. Yet all of these conditions—and many more—can be caused/worsened by the microwave radiation from wireless devices. Many hospitals are now introducing the use of wireless tablets to assess and report on a patient's health, seemingly oblivious to the impact of this device on the body of someone who is already ill or in a weakened state. Most hospitals also have WiFi throughout their facilities, permeating every ward, including the ICU, where patients may be recovering from brain surgery for the removal of a tumour caused by this same WiFi radiation. Using the cause of the problem to try to override or address the problem is the ultimate irony in a world that's so full of ironies that people no longer see what's right in front of them. So focused are they on getting their wireless fix that they can't see what that device is doing to their health, their brains, their social skills or their lives.

9. Your radiation-scrambled brain may not be able to process the fact that it has been scrambled. The brain-scrambling effect of microwave radiation often prevents us from registering the fact that our brain has been affected. It therefore prevents us from processing that reality or from finding a way to remove ourselves from further harm. This phenomenon makes microwaves one of the most insidious and effective means of disabling or dumbing-down those affected by it. The only way to minimize this effect is to somehow train yourself to immediately leave any environment in which your brain starts to feel sluggish and you have difficulty thinking clearly or keeping your balance. If you have a partner, ask him or her to watch out for the signs of this brain-scrambling effect and to help you get to a safer place if you are affected.

10. You may feel like a victim, but it all comes down to you. While man-made electromagnetic radiation may affect you so severely that it tears your life apart, try to see beyond what's happening on the surface. The challenges of being electro-sensitive go far beyond our physical or mental well-being. They are, in fact, a push to empowerment. They represent the ultimate wake-up call, alerting us to the fact that we have lost touch with who we really are, as electromagnetic beings, and what we need to do to stay healthy, balanced and in harmony with our environment. We are being called upon to recognize the fundamental flaws in our fast-paced, gadget-driven existence and to tap into our higher faculties to create a truly healthy, sustainable reality. Although we need to speak out against those who harm us, and to make healthier boundaries in order to reclaim our autonomy and self-respect, we must go beyond merely ranting and raving at the authorities. If you've been physically backed into a corner, with nowhere else to go but inside yourself, *go there*—for that is where you will find true freedom. It's not about letting the wireless industry/ governments off the hook. It's about recognizing how the current situation has led to your internal power being suppressed and needing to be activated; it's about understanding the nature of your electromagnetism and how to make it work for you; and it's about tapping into your higher faculties to literally change your situation from the inside out—using the neuroplasticity of your brain, the quantum laws of the universe, and your unique creative capacity to transform your physical reality. Having microwave sickness or electro-sensitivity is not about what's been done to you, beyond your control; it's about taking back control of your self, your body and your life. It's about mastering your mind and body in ways that put you back in touch with what it means to be divinely human and to live in respectful harmony with your natural world. It's about getting *truly* connected—not via a cell phone, but with your heart and your deeper spiritual self, and with the hearts, minds and spirits of your fellow human beings.

PART 4
THE CALL TO CONSCIOUSNESS

51 Are you dodging the call?

We are all called to greatness in different ways. Crises, illness, personal loss and financial debt are just some of the ways that we are challenged to tap into some deeper part of ourselves to find a higher way forward and to become more empowered in our own lives. Some of us willingly heed that call, while others resist or remain unaware of it, continuing to operate the way they have always operated—trying harder and harder to make things work, yet getting the same mixed results as before.

Being affected by electromagnetic radiation is just one doorway to wholeness and one way we may be called to activate the greatness that resides within us all. It almost doesn't matter which door you choose (none of them are winners). You could choose the doorway of disease, of climate change or of economic collapse. But they would all take you to the same place, provided you had your eyes open going through that door. Choose Door 1, Door 2 or Door 3, and you'll end up with same underlying drivers of the problem: human dysfunction due to limiting beliefs and a distorted perception of self and how the world works.

Why do we resist our greatness? Why do we dodge the call? We have become so conditioned to believe that the problems are 'out there', rather than being taught that we are the creators of the scenarios that we call life. And, in believing that our problems come from outside of us, we naturally try to address them in the same way, often blaming those external parties who appear to be responsible for what is happening to us.

I've done a lot of artful dodging in my time—and getting a brain tumour from microwave radiation was not my first wake-up call. In the early 90s, when I initially began to explore spirituality and the impact of our subconscious programming on our lives, I was seeking answers to some chronic health issues and I was already being affected by EMFs, without realizing it. Despite developing and teaching some powerful tools for self-mastery, however, I did not embrace them as fully as I could have. Clearly, I needed a much bigger and more arresting wake-up call to push me past my own resistance. More accurately, that event caused much of my knowledge to come back up to the surface and to make me conscious of just how much had remained beyond my awareness. But knowing something is not the same as embodying it and I had yet to actively apply some of the principles that I intellectually knew to be valid.

Say YES to greatness. Don't dodge the call.
There's too much at stake and we all need you AWAKE!

Ironically, when we begin to understand the true source of our circumstances and start to take responsibility for them, we undergo a process that's similar to what we experience when we lose someone we love. First described by Dr Elisabeth Kübler-Ross in her book *On Death and Dying* (1969), the five stages of grief mirror the emotions we feel when we let go of the old self. Even though we never unconditionally loved the person that we were (which had many layers of conditioning and was influenced more by others than by our own true self), we resist letting it go because we have invested so much in the old way of thinking and behaving. Even when we consciously choose to let go of the old self, we usually find ourselves experiencing those five stages of grief: denial, anger, bargaining, depression and acceptance.

When I think of the EMF situation, I can see how these emotions kicked in as I tried to address things:

1. I was in denial about the harm being caused and didn't want to believe it, at first.

2. I experienced anger when my voice went unheard and nothing was done.

3. I tried to negotiate (bargain) with those harming me.

4. I became deeply depressed—about the losses sustained by our natural environment and by me personally, during those years of my life when I was only half living.

5. I experienced acceptance of self and of the deeper truth as I remembered the power of me.

"When you learn your lessons, the pain goes away."

—Dr Elisabeth Kübler-Ross

Only then, in fact, did I really start to address the issue of EMFs in a meaningful way. I had to completely let go of the old way of doing this. I had to stop my mind from dwelling on the injustices and from coming up with clever strategies for launching another attack on my aggressors. This meant disengaging from those who were still focused on what was happening 'out there', as opposed to tapping into the power within. It meant letting go of the need to be right, which is something that has been deeply engrained in me for as long as I can remember. Initially, it felt as if I was giving up and allowing the other side to win. After all, I was withdrawing from the ring and no longer willing to throw any more punches. But the wiser part of me knew that the other side was not winning at all. It might look as if it was, but there is no 'win' if our environment is being harmed. No one wins if it's at the expense of someone else. That's not a 'win'; it's a suppression of those in a temporarily weakened state who are being pushed to reclaim their autonomy and take back the power they unwittingly gave away.

The wireless telecoms industry and our industry-driven governments are mere sparring partners who reflect the weaknesses in our attack and the need for a completely different approach.

52 Creators and curators: we are both

Addressing the multi-faceted issue of our EMF-polluted world requires a multi-dimensional approach that goes beyond creative thinking, clever marketing and hard-hitting campaigns. Our environmental impact is now so extensive and pervasive that we must dig far deeper into ourselves to access and apply the full spectrum of human resources at our disposal.

Although it serves us to think creatively in all that we do, we have a far greater impact when we think of ourselves as *creators*. This means that we don't just use our minds to come up with a new approach; we must consciously tap into the universal mind and the quantum field, leveraging our phenomenal powers of perception and intentionality to cultivate the desired outcome. If we also see ourselves as *curators*—the temporary guardians and custodians of our precious planetary home—we shift from mindless consumption to conscious gratitude for all that we've been gifted. And gratitude, as Dr Joe Dispenza so eloquently puts it, is the ultimate form of receivership. Plus, the longer we linger in gratitude, he says, the more we draw our new life to us.[100]

We must consciously leverage our phenomenal powers of perception and intentionality to cultivate the desired outcome.

Being grateful for our capacity to create and curate is therefore an essential part of manifesting whatever outcome we desire, since gratitude makes us magnets for more of what we love. If we actively love ourselves by respecting our bodies' physical, emotional and spiritual needs, we demonstrate gratitude for who and what we are, while also embodying healthy self-worth, which has its own powerful magnetism.

We have all the skills and faculties we need to be endlessly creative, and we have a responsibility to create and evolve in harmony with our planetary home. (Being passive consumers, feeding off the planet without contributing in a meaningful way to sustain the necessary healthy balance, is not what we came here to do.) When we receive an inspiring, creative idea (downloaded to us from universal intelligence—no wireless microwave devices required!), we must, as creators and curators, treat it like a newborn that we are privileged to conceive, nourish and deliver into the world. It is gifted to us, just like the air that we breathe.

Yet, due to conditioning, it's sometimes difficult for us to have faith in ourselves and to trust in the universe to support and facilitate whatever endeavour we might undertake, with the right energy. We often fail to trust that our needs will be met and that we don't have to struggle to make things work. That's true for anyone who has been programmed to believe that they must work hard to survive or succeed—and that belief alone will determine how easy or hard life is, whether we're dealing with EMFs or a creative project.

I spent years in victim mode, after getting a tumour, convinced that I was powerless to change things. Now that I'm transitioning back to a more empowered way of thinking and behaving, there is bound to be some resistance from my deeply engrained programs (and my big fat ego), trying to pull me back into the old paradigm of reactivity. Even if I'm not conscious of my own resistance, Lewis always reflects back to me my deeper issues. He is my greatest mirror, trigger and teacher, generating more ideas and creative thinking (plus a few meltdowns) than I would otherwise have experienced if he'd always been completely in agreement with me. How boring would *that* be?

We all need mirrors to reflect what we are doing ... or failing to do. Yet the whole world is our mirror, with various people, dynamics and circumstances sending us very powerful messages about what's going on inside. It would be nice to have a magic mirror that interpreted our circumstances for us so we could get instant feedback about what's really going on.

Mirror, mirror, on the wall, what's the EMFing point of it all?

Whether you're launching a creative project or trying to find a creative solution to the issue of EMFs in your environment, you must give your idea room to breathe and grow. Ideas need to be able to gain some creative momentum, before having a structure imposed on them, so that they can generate the right energy for connecting with the right people in the right way. I sometimes feel a crushing disappointment if I present an idea to Lewis too early in that process, and he immediately wants to implement a strategy or a plan. I can feel the heavy weight of control dragging the idea down to the level of our three-dimensional reality. That's not where magic happens. It happens in our hearts and out there, in the quantum field, where all things are possible. Yet once an idea has matured and grown in the right kind of energy, structured delivery mechanisms can give it the wings it needs to take off.

Creativity is the most potent enlivener of all our endeavours, whether we're dealing with a personal project or addressing the challenges of EMFs. It is the essential leavening agent in all our greatest human recipes, raising our frequency to a higher dimension of possibility. Without it, we grapple with mere mechanics, implementing a system, pushing paper from here to there, or trying to convince, persuade or cajole through words or actions alone. If our efforts lack a creative spark, or fail to be fuelled by gratitude and universal intelligence (our most powerful ally in creating the outcomes we seek), we may find ourselves struggling to make things work.

Creativity is the essential leavening agent in all our greatest human recipes, raising our frequency to a higher dimension of possibility.

In the same way that we do not own our children, we do not own our ideas. They come to us, often unbidden, and we provide the vehicle for their delivery. We must feed and nourish them, allowing them to lead and inspire us until they are ready to take off. In reality, *they* feed *us*, enlivening us with their creative spark and the very energy of creation. With every idea that comes to us, we have the opportunity to either demonstrate our capacity for creation or reinforce our limiting beliefs. The issue of EMFs provides the same opportunity, yet many of us are stuck at the fork in the road, not realizing that we can choose greatness over defeat. It's a dichotomy that exists throughout our existence—a duality of evolutionary paths that offers us, in every moment, the option of choosing the higher road.

Whatever idea or goal you might have, whether it's for a business or for resolving the issue of EMFs in your life, it must be supported by five key elements in order for it to fly.

1. An unshakable faith in yourself and in your entitlement to health, happiness and fulfillment.

2. A clear vision, energized by an uplifting emotion such as excitement, passion or love.

3. A deep abiding gratitude, as if your vision is already a reality.

4. Thoughts, words and actions that align with your positive intent and with healthy self-worth.

5. A connection with universal intelligence (through meditation, yoga or stillness) and a sense of responsibility, purpose and delight for your role in creating the life you want.

53

No, you can't! A mantra for the can-do digital age

Ten years ago, when former US President Barack Obama made his rallying post-election cry—*Yes, you can!*—I heard it as a call to empowerment. *Yes, you can have a better life. Yes, you can make a difference.* In our self-serving modern society, however, our sense of entitlement seems to have become overblown. In this digital age, we believe we can have and do anything we want. *I can, so I will.* With unlimited worldwide access to information and resources, geographical boundaries have dissolved, and so have most of our personal ones.

We've become used to hearing YES—YES to more data-download capacity, to faster Internet speeds, to competitive prices, to buying whatever we want, to accessing whatever information we seek, to having all the latest gadgets, to getting instant responses to e-mails, and to living the good life in the fast lane. We don't want to hear NO. If we hear a NO, we look for a way around it. *How much does a YES cost?* Whatever we want, we will find a way to get it.

Are you selfie-centred?

In our selfie-centred culture, even those who have documented the dangers of electromagnetic radiation make a point of telling people that they don't have to give up their smartphone, mobile connectivity or wireless gadgets. Instead, they cater to the collective dependence, suggesting ways for users to reduce their exposure and to make their bodies more resilient against all the ambient radiation. The focus is on the all-important *consumer*. But what about the impact of EMR on plants, crops, animals, insects, the environment and the climate? What about the planet on which we depend for our survival? Giving consumers what they want does not factor in the cost of YES. The number of people dependent on their wireless gadgets is now so vast that no one wants to say NO to them—perhaps because they themselves are equally gadget-dependent, because they have a vested interest in sustaining that dependence, or because they are afraid of being rejected for challenging the status quo.

In conversation with someone who had regained her health after years of illness due to multiple chemical sensitivity and electro-sensitivity, I asked what she felt had helped her. Many things, she said, but one of the most significant factors was that she learned to say NO—NO to over-extending herself, to living in a toxic environment, to pleasing others and to putting others' needs before her own.

When NO to others = YES to you

In my counselling practice, I encourage people to say YES to healthy self-acceptance, healthy self-care and wise choices, and to say NO to unhealthy compromises, abuse and self-neglect. We have become confused in our priorities. We seem to think that saying YES to convenience, to having high-tech gadgets and to doing what we want, whenever we want, is equivalent to saying YES to ourselves in generous, positive ways. But it is not a healthy, loving YES or a sustainable one.

We must start saying NO. We tell young people to say NO to drugs, yet we bombard them with harmful radiation. We say NO to child abuse, yet we daily abuse our children by irradiating their vulnerable brains and bodies. We say NO to animal vivisection and cruelty, yet we subject wildlife and all life forms to deadly emissions from our high-tech gadgets. Healthcare practitioners (even many naturopaths) tell us to eat better, exercise more and take better care of our health ...yet they use all kinds of wireless devices in their office, where we go to get well.

If this wireless technology is here to stay, it will outlive us.

NO is currently the most vital yet under-used, life-saving word in our vocabulary. If we don't start saying NO to more and YES to less, we will drown in our own indulgent dysfunction. We must stop behaving like spoiled rich kids with sophisticated toys that we refuse to give up. As we recognize the need to become conscious of what our actions are costing the planet, applying the *power of no* becomes even more critical. No, you can't roll out 5G, because it's going to ultimately cause mass extinctions. No, you can't put WiFi in schools, because it fries young brains and bodies, causing sickness, despair, genetic damage and suicides. No, you can't have a cell phone; you're only 3 years old. No, you can't go online while we're having dinner. No, you can't do whatever you want just because you are physically able to.

We seem to be as afraid of now—of being present—as we are of NO. We may be afraid of losing friends, of being rejected or of being seen as *not nice* if we fail to accommodate others' needs, even if doing so hurts us. But those kinds of unhealthy compromises say as much about our own shaky self-worth as they do about the kind of company we keep (with one feeding the other, unless we break the unhealthy cycle).

No, you can't! In an age of limitless possibilities, this must become our new mantra if we are to have healthy boundaries with our children, partners, gadget-loving friends, or any government/industry that violates our right to live in a healthy environment.

Cultivating personal boundaries begins at home, and the more we embody healthy boundaries at the personal level—with ourselves, our friends, our partners and our family—the more we naturally enforce them with our colleagues, our bosses, and anyone else in a position of apparent authority. Ironically, the more we do this, the more authority we emanate and the more respect we command from others.

Let's say YES to healthy behaviour on all levels, and NO to whatever fails to support our healthy evolution on this planet. We don't need anyone's permission to say NO to what's harmful, and we already have the right—and the responsibility—to say YES to your own healthy autonomy.

Yes, we can do this.

54

From microwave to macrowave: creating a tsunami of consciousness

When we understand the tremendous impact and benefits of being fully conscious, spiritually active and empowered, we are motivated to live differently. We nourish ourselves better. We let go of meaningless 'stuff' and clutter. We gravitate towards nature, stillness and meditation. We embrace and explore our innate creativity. We're discerning in the company we keep and the conversations we have. We recognize our role as creators and the need to live consciously. We cultivate a state of perpetual receivership, through gratitude and self-acceptance. We sense our interconnectedness and our multi-dimensional nature. And we know we can change our world from the inside out.

When we do all these things—effectively clearing and enlightening our system, boosting our personal electromagnetic field, and consciously tapping into the quantum field of infinite possibilities—there is nothing we cannot accomplish. Instead of being electronically enslaved, drama-driven or convenience-addicted in a world that has lost its connection to what matters most, we activate our humanity, connecting to our hearts and souls ...and to each other.

**Technology keeps us focused on externals
rather than tapping into our creatorship.**

The worldwide obsession with perpetual connectivity reflects our deep yearning for a spiritual connection with ourselves, with nature and with each other. Technology will never bring us happiness or true fulfillment. It merely distracts us from what's missing within, keeping us focused on externals rather than tapping in to our creatorship. All the ills of our modern era come from this loss of consciousness—a disconnection from who we really are and what we are here to do.

Addressing the impact of EMFs in our environment represents a global opportunity for us to heal our planet. Even if governments are ultimately forced to acknowledge and address the widespread harm caused by electromagnetic radiation, the deeper issues will remain. Our lack of personal and planetary responsibility will not have been addressed and we will continue to be the victims of those to whom we have ceded our authority.

The effects of EMFs offer many insights for those who wish to look deeper and take responsibility for what's happening. They serve as the indicators of what we need to address within, since the actions of industry/government/service-providers are a direct reflection of what we are doing to ourselves. In fact, it's only *because* of our actions/inaction that the 'authorities' can do what they're doing, with apparent impunity.

So, what *are* they doing? They are violating our rights and boundaries, disrespecting us and our choices, disregarding our health, overloading our bodies with harmful stuff, being inconsiderate of our needs, putting money/convenience/profit over all else, and generally behaving in an unconscious, unenlightened way. Yet haven't we all done these very same things to ourselves and others—and aren't we still doing them? Do we not violate personal boundaries every day—in our interactions with our partners, colleagues or other drivers on the road? Do we not routinely abuse, overload and/or over-extend our bodies, through bad food choices, stress or other means? Don't we all make unhealthy compromises for the sake of acceptance, money, convenience or advancement?

We have done to ourselves and to each other everything that we now see the industry/government doing to us. Can we then, in all integrity, claim that what industry/government is doing to us is unacceptable? Are we not embodying double standards that send mixed messages to almost every 'unhealthy' industry, giving tacit permission for them to treat us the way we treat ourselves?

Through our actions and choices, we let them know what our needs and priorities are, and they're just giving us what we've asked for:

I want to be well but I want a quick fix, so I'd prefer to take a pill instead of figuring out why I'm sick.

I don't like the idea of radiation affecting me, but I want better coverage for my phone as I need it for my work, friends etc.

I need to eat better but I don't have time to cook so I'll get a TV dinner/pizza/pre-cooked meal.

I'm over-worked, stressed, unloved and unhappy, but social media makes me feel better so I need to be online at least six hours a day, wherever I am.

If we see this dynamic as a reflection of what we need to address within ourselves, we can reclaim our autonomy, while consciously healing and empowering ourselves. In so doing, we will heal far more than our individual bodies, since empowering ourselves has an impact at the quantum level, far beyond our physical form.

"To be healthy in today's world,
you need to access and cultivate a reliance on yourself."

—Dr Kelly Brogan, MD, in *A Mind of Your Own*

We can change our minds about who we are and what we can achieve. We can change our perception of how the world works. We can intentionally direct our thoughts to produce a positive external effect. We can make new choices that support the environment we want to create. When we make those shifts, everything changes. But we must first accept that we are responsible for our own situations. All the clues we need to fix the sickness in our world are inherent in our own behaviour and in whatever we feel is missing in our lives.

Collective empowerment is the only thing that will create the tsunami of consciousness needed to restore balance in our bodies and our environment. But it's not just about healing our bodies or leading a healthier lifestyle. It's about graduating to a whole new level of self-awareness, intentionality and spiritual connectedness that enables us to go far beyond our usual way of perceiving and resolving problems.

55 Setting your intention

Even if we know what needs to be done to protect ourselves and our planet, we often seem to resist doing it. The majority of us don't consciously *want* to evolve. Mostly, we want outcomes—more money, better job, loving relationship, nice house—but that's not evolution. It's usually more about us acquiring or achieving things by striving for them with hard work and good intentions. And it's largely unconscious, with our early conditioning driving our behaviour, while also causing us to attract a reflection of whatever beliefs we embody. You think life is tough and that there's no free lunch? Your subconscious mind will reflect that back to you, bringing you ample evidence (in the form of circumstances) that this is exactly the way life is. Such is the power of you, with your electrically charged thoughts and your magnetic feelings attracting exactly what you transmit.

To the extent that most of us underestimate the power of all the man-made electromagnetic fields in our external environment, we also underestimate the power of our own electromagnetism.

The powerful impact of environmental electromagnetic fields (EMFs) is designed to put us in touch with our internal EMFs. Those of us seeking to raise awareness of the dangers or to push governments to take action already know that the alarm calls are not being heeded, yet we don't always perceive the deeper truth beneath this frustrating failure to act (theirs or ours). And the general lack of consciousness about both forms of EMFs is taking us on a downward spiral. We are misguidedly increasing man-made frequencies while failing to increase our own natural frequencies, thereby creating a 'double whammy'.

**We currently stand at the crossroads between
self-annihilation and greatness.**

Only one thing will bring us out of this nosedive: consciousness, driven by a true desire to evolve as humans, rather than by proxy, via our electronic gadgets. Evolution is about tapping into our higher faculties and operating

246

from a place of true creation—making something from nothing—so that what transpires in our lives is the result of us consciously utilizing our own internal electromagnetism to create true fulfillment.

Not wanting to evolve is the same thing as not wanting to be conscious, since one would automatically lead to the other. This is where we currently stand: at the crossroads between self-annihilation and greatness.

If we become conscious, we see our greatness …and maybe that's what scares some of us, since we've been so deeply programmed to NOT be powerful. Yet that programming (limiting beliefs we have about who we are and what's possible) is really the only thing that stops us from wholeheartedly embracing consciousness with exuberance and delight for the magic we can create. If we catch a glimpse of that magic within ourselves, we may be inspired to go further; but if we've lived our lives with no concept of our phenomenal creative powers or the support that's available to us from universal intelligence, there would be no reason to get excited about the possibilities. Even reading about this kind of thing might be annoying, if we have no frame of reference for such power.

The wireless telecoms industry and governments are denying the power of their EMFs, just as we are denying the power of ours. And, in the same way that they deny the solid scientific evidence of that powerful impact, most of us tend to deny or minimize the scientific validity of quantum physics and neuroscience, once we become aware of it. In reality, such denial reflects our lack of faith in ourselves to exert enough influence to change things. Yet we have that power and it resides in our thoughts, words, behaviour and feelings.

> "[W]hen a thought activates a molecule in the brain,
> it is actually performing a quantum operation."
>
> —Dr Deepak Chopra, in *The Quantum Doctor*, by Amit Goswami

Quantum physicists have demonstrated beyond any doubt that our thoughts have an impact on our world. While we may nonetheless be tempted to justify our apparent insignificance, telling ourselves that we cannot compete with such formidable adversaries is no longer valid. If we choose to continue justifying our apparent inability to make a difference, we are as much in denial about our power to create a positive impact as the industry is in denial about its negative impact on our world.

Given the state of our microwaved environment and given your power as an electromagnetic individual, what is your intention? Who and what do you intend to be, given your undeniable capacity to change things for the better? Do you intend to allow things to continue as they are, or will you choose to focus your thoughts and feelings on creating the world you ideally want?

Intention + attention = a force for change

Just like everything else in the universe, our thoughts are energy, and they can be measured as electrical wave patterns in the brain. "[L]ike any other set of particles or source of energy, we are entangled with everything we've ever encountered, the environment around us and the rest of the universe," says investigative journalist Peter Baksa.[101]

Because we are conscious, we can choose what part of the randomness around us to be affected by, he says, and how we in turn would like to affect it. It is through the property of entanglement that we can effect change in our environment. "Our minds are transceivers, able to receive and send signals into the 'quantum soup' [...] by way of the highly coherent frequencies of our thoughts."

The higher the frequency of our thought/brain wave, the higher our consciousness, Baksa explains. The level of our consciousness is what makes our reality what it is and what it will continue to be.

We have the power to change whatever we decide we have the power to change. Once we grasp the phenomenal power of human consciousness, and when we understand our electromagnetism, we begin to see our greatness. We start to take responsibility for ourselves because we know we are in charge. Then, when we engage with the quantum field and feed a positive intention for the future, we can literally create the kind of healthy environment and empowered living that will leave all our wireless gadgets in the shade.

Feed your vision of the future

First, define your vision. What does it look and feel like? What kind of healthy environment, vibrant lifestyle or emotional freedom do you envision? What qualities and emotions make up that vision? How do you feel in that envisioned future reality? Give it as much feeling, colour and life as you can.

Then ask yourself what feeds that vision. In every single choice that you make, ask yourself if doing or not doing that particular thing will feed or detract from your vision. Be mindful of your thoughts and words, adjusting them so that they support and nourish your emerging reality. Remember that every thought, word and action has a vibration that ripples out into your world to create an effect.

Get excited and be deeply grateful for your ideal future reality (no matter how seemingly implausible), as if it already exists. This generates very powerful energy and magnetism into the quantum field, where your envisioned reality will take shape.

Regularly meditating will help you to quieten your mind, create stillness in your body, boost your intentionality, and sharpen your focus. Think of your vision as a powerful beam of energy shooting out into the universe. The more focused and mindful we are, the more present we are, and being present is the key to processing life and creating what we desire. Being present keeps us connected to our feelings (which guide our choices) and to what is going on inside and 'around us, while preventing us from sinking into the numbness that comes from being emotionally overwhelmed and spiritually disconnected.

In order to realize whatever vision we might have, we must cultivate an elevated state of consciousness so that we connect with universal intelligence and its infinite possibilities. As Dr Amit Goswami says in his book, *The Quantum Doctor*, we have the capacity to choose our own reality. However, to do so, "we need to be in a non-ordinary state of 'illumined' consciousness".[102]

The more we cultivate this enlightened state, the more connected we feel, the more powerfully we can realize our vision or goals, and the more peace we experience in our lives. In the same way that we must build physical muscle in order to do push-ups, we must work our spiritual muscles if we are to become more spiritually connected and attuned. With a regular meditation practice, we develop a sense of being connected to everything and each other—a feeling of oneness that people experience when they meditate regularly. In the same way that the oceans are all connected, we too are connected through the air that we breathe. And just as my electromagnetic field radiates out into the space around me, your electromagnetic field radiates out into the space around you, with all of us overlapping, even if we're not aware of this happening. As we work our spiritual 'muscles', we develop greater awareness of ourselves, of the energy in and around us, and of our interconnectedness.

The following seven-step process may help you to cultivate greater consciousness so you can fulfill your vision of vibrant health, emotional/physical freedom and joyful living, or whatever you envision.

1. **Create a quiet, comfortable, private space where you can focus.** Eliminate any distractions or noise.

2. **Focus on your breath** and begin to breathe deeply and slowly, consciously relaxing your body with every exhale. Choose to let go of thoughts and concerns, and focus on the space between your thoughts.

3. **Become aware of your body sitting in stillness** and allow any feelings and thoughts to just pass through you, always returning your focus to the breath and to the space between your thoughts.

4. **Try to connect with your heart** and send yourself and others loving thoughts. Think of the compassion and love you feel for those close

to you. Visualize these feelings radiating out from your heart into the universe, creating a field of uplifting, healing energy.

5. **Envision your ideal future reality** and see it as vividly as you can. Engage all of your senses and experience that reality as if it already exists, feeling the joy, excitement and fulfillment of living that reality now.

6. **Feel your heart swell with gratitude for this new reality.** Dwell in deep gratitude for as long as you can, knowing that being grateful for everything you love brings you more of the same.

7. **Keep this feeling with you** as you slowly come back to the present moment and re-engage with your day. Allow this feeling to guide your thoughts, words and actions so that they feed, and are in alignment with, your vision and keep you emotionally and spiritually connected to it.

If we truly want our vision or intention to manifest in physical form, we must take responsibility for the choices we make in our everyday lives. No matter how much we might want vibrant health, a pristine environment or the freedom to go/do whatever we want, our vision is unlikely to materialise unless we stay true to our intention. As always, the universe will bring us whatever (or more of whatever) we are putting our attention on. We must therefore take full responsibility for whatever shows up, since it is the direct result of our focus and whatever we are transmitting consistently enough to produce that particular outcome.

We must also trust in our own wisdom, in the power of our intention, and in what we know to be true about ourselves, while trusting in the evidence provided by quantum physics about how the world really works.

56 Decoding the crisis and coming back to life

When we understand the nature of the crisis and what it represents, we get a sense of what we are being called upon to do as individuals, in our own lives. Wherever there is dysfunction, the challenge usually lies in doing the opposite of what we have been doing—or the opposite of whatever is being done to us that we do not like. In other words, we must embody whatever healthy, positive, life-enhancing qualities are missing from our lives.

If you want to be free—emotionally free to make conscious wise choices and to create the life you desire—you must clear out old negative programs and stories, nourish and energize your body, spend time in nature, and engage your spirit. If you don't consciously want that degree of freedom, avoid doing anything that will stir things up and you will be able to hang on to all your cherished beliefs and convictions. You won't be lonely, either, as lots of people prefer not to change or to take responsibility for their own lives. You may not be healthy or happy, and it's unlikely that you'll manifest your ideal life or environment, but you'll be in familiar territory, which can sometimes seem preferable to the unknown. Only you can decide. Ultimately, though, we are all pushed to be powerful, whether we consciously want to be or not.

Consciousness checklist: are you conscious enough to want to be fully conscious?

If you are serious about taking responsibility for yourself and for the global situation we have all created, think about what you are transmitting to your world and those around you. Consider how much your lifestyle and choices deplete or contribute to our planetary resources, and think about what you are ready and willing to change.

- Would you complain if you had to get out of bed or walk a few feet to answer your corded phone instead of reaching for your cordless/cell phone? Or do you give thanks for your awareness and your ability to protect your health?

- Do you get frustrated if you don't get good cell phone coverage when you're trying to make a call? Or are you glad to have a healthy space and some quiet time to yourself to focus on what's in front of you?

- Using a cell phone feeds the demand for more cell towers and more radiation. Is that what you want to do? You can justify your choices in terms of what you 'need' for your work etc, but there's no negotiating with nature. Either we're treating our environment respectfully or we're not—and it's already clear that we've made far too many choices that suit our needs at the expense of our natural resources.

- How much time do you spend on your computer, iPad, cell phone or other means of online connectivity? What is this doing to your brain, your nervous system, your social skills and your ability to concentrate? How is it changing you as a person? If you can't tear yourself away from an e-mail or text when a real person tries to talk to you, what does this tell you?

- What does it say about you, your values, your self-worth, your personal boundaries and your relationships if you feel the need to have your cell phone beside you at all times, wherever you go, even in a restaurant while having an intimate dinner with your spouse/partner? What message are you giving them about their importance in your life?

- Do you have healthy boundaries around the time you spend online? Do you have healthy limits in terms of the foods you eat? Do you put yourself first, in healthy ways? What unhealthy compromises do you make with others, in the hope of some wished-for outcome?

- In what ways do you over-extend yourself? (Admit it. You do!)

- Do you smoke to de-stress, take pharmaceutical/recreational drugs to treat symptoms, eat processed foods/sugar for comfort, use alcohol to unwind, drink coffee to get going, take sleeping pills to sleep, or stay up too late because you're over-stimulated? Take a moment to ask yourself why you do any/all of these things. There is a reason for everything we do; we might be able to hide the truth from ourselves for a while (aka living in denial), but our unresolved issues and addictions ultimately backfire.

- If you spend hours online and your cell phone is stuck to your body like a limpet, are you willing to acknowledge being addicted to social media and non-stop connectivity, thereby feeding this unhealthy, destructive lifestyle? And are you willing to explore the deeper drivers of this addiction, the impacts of your behaviour, and what you can do to create more deeply rewarding and meaningful human interactions?

- How many parallels do you see between the way you treat yourself and the way industry/government treats you?

- In what ways might you be supporting whatever industry you feel is harming you?

A lack of healthy self-worth—and the resulting lack of conscious self-care—has impacts far beyond what we might see in our immediate environment. If we lived with greater self-respect, self-acceptance and self-responsibility, we would never reach this point of global dysfunction, disconnectedness and disease. What we do to our bodies, we do to our planet—and all major corporations and industries take full advantage of the unmet needs and addictions that promote the crucial imbalance, inside and out.

Our growing disconnectedness ensures the continued existence of the countless industries that feed our need for some kind of 'surrogate' product or service that will (we hope) help us feel better about ourselves. But co-dependence never works long term, and there is no substitute for the real thing—the kind of conscious human connection that provides the love and fulfillment we all seek.

57 EMF off! day: freedom from e-slavery

By the end of 2017, an estimated 300 million people worldwide were feeling the effects of the man-made electromagnetic radiation in our environment. Many of those individuals may feel powerless against the massive telecoms industry and its progressive assault on our health, our human rights and our planet. Yet if 300 million people healed and empowered themselves, collectively focusing on the healthy environment they wished to create, inside and out, can you imagine the impact we would have?

Together, we are more powerful than any industry on Earth. It is merely our lack of *awareness* of our power that keeps us stuck in subservience. Recognizing, embracing and activating our creatorship is the most powerful and effective thing we can do to create the world we want. The devastating impact of EMFs is pushing us to the limits of our tolerance, and it is time to push back with everything we've got. If we do this together, we will be unstoppable. We will be amazed and gratified by our global impact. We will fall in love with ourselves and our planet, and we will be committed to ensuring that both are protected, honoured and respected, for the benefit of all.

I am therefore launching an EMF off! day, to be celebrated every year on 25 March, which is also the International Day of Remembrance of the Victims of Slavery, endorsed by the United Nations.[103] We have been enslaved for far too long—enslaved to technology, to governments, and to our own dysfunction—and it's time to break free. On this commemorative day, we can remind ourselves of who we really are. We can switch off our electronic devices (wired or otherwise) and instead connect in person with each other, our neighbours, our friends, our family and nature. Fittingly, this day comes after the International Day for the Right to the Truth Concerning Gross Human Rights Violations and for the Dignity of Victims (on 24 March). Reclaiming our autonomy and reclaiming our rights are one and the same, and we have the power and the responsibility to do both.

If we stay stuck in subservience, reacting to external circumstances rather than creating the circumstances we want, we do each other a great disservice. We compound our dysfunction and reinforce our position as victims, adding to the problem rather than being part of the solution. Let's not do that any more. Let's unite in empowerment rather than in victimhood, and in promoting the good news rather than the bad. Let's share our stories of empowerment and success, rather than dwelling on or reinforcing our failure to have a meaningful impact. Let's remind each other of our power as creators, rather than affirming what hasn't worked. Let's get ourselves switched on, fully activated in our humanity and fully empowered in the way we live. We owe it to each other to embody the change we want to see, when greatness beckons and our planet is at risk.

What you can do on EMF off! day

- **Switch off from technology and switch on your humanity.** Connect with family, friends and neighbours and be truly present, giving them your fullest attention, with no cell phones, computers or other distractions diluting your focus in the moment. Bring someone a gift, talk to people on the street and have a conscious conversation, really listening to what's being said.

- **Reduce the demand that you have helped to create.** There is no industry on Earth that can survive unless we feed the demand for it. Likewise, if there is a demand for a healthier alternative, someone will invent a less harmful technology. Find a way to reduce your dependence on the wireless industry …and keep looking for eco-friendly alternatives. Switch from a smartphone to a flip phone, to be used only for essential calls. Do all other work and data downloads on a wired computer. It may be inconvenient, but so is cancer, which doesn't come with an OFF switch.

- **Reduce your ambient EMFs and boost your own electromagnetic field.** Laughter, music, creativity, meditation, yoga and being in nature boost your electromagnetic field and nourish your spirit. The body thrives when nourished in these simple ways, all of which counter the negative effects of sitting at a computer, commuting to work or living in a high-rise building. Play with your dog, earth your body by lying on the grass, notice the trees and the changing season, look up at the sky, move your body and give your mind a rest.

- **Wire and inspire.** There are many benefits to having your computer hardwired, beyond the health-related ones. Keeping your computer/laptop in your office or other designated workspace creates a healthy boundary between your virtual world and your real one. This enhances your relationships, your capacity to be emotionally present, and the importance you give to those close to you. By 'closing the door' on that other world of endless distractions, you immediately become more emotionally and physically available—to yourself as well as to others. In sharing more of yourself, you will inspire others to do the same.

- **Pay attention to what you have neglected.** What aspects of your self have you neglected or allowed to become dormant, while focusing on work, e-mails, texts or social media? If there's some challenge in your life, go for a walk and let your mind ponder some creative solutions instead of looking for instant answers online. In being electronically on, what have you not done for yourself? Buy yourself a plant. Go for a massage. Move your body. Cook an elaborate, delicious meal, using healthy organic ingredients and your own imagination. Read a book.

- **Slow down and stop multi-tasking.** We are all moving so fast that we rarely give ourselves a chance to process things or integrate life. Allow your mind to catch up and life will flow more smoothly.

- **Do nothing.** Sit in stillness, allow your body and mind to be peaceful, and give yourself a chance to get good at it. You will then be less likely to crave distractions or to depend on social media or other online interactions in the hope of creating a meaningful connection.

58 Where do you begin?

As I lie on the deck in the wintry January sunshine, clothed from head to toe, with my face the only 'vitamin D porthole' for the sun's healing rays to enter, I reflect on all that has happened. Looking up at the cloudless sky, I wonder, as always, *where does the blue begin?* Given all that I have learned, it's a question that prompts several others: Where do *we* begin? When will *you* begin? Where and how do we start being powerfully, uncompromisingly our true selves?

Before we explore and activate our higher faculties, we can take practical steps to boost our sense of self and to create a wholesome living environment. Whether we have been harmed by EMFs and forced into a defensive position, or we have been harmed by personal experiences and relationships, these steps will help us to create healthier dynamics and boundaries in our lives. Once we have created this solid foundation, we will be better equipped to explore our spiritual and co-creative capacities.

A two-pronged approach to healing

Regaining our autonomy and humanity requires reclaiming the most essential parts of ourselves that we have lost: our voice, our self-responsibility and our spiritual sovereignty. It also means separating ourselves from the environment that harmed us and from the story in which we became disconnected, so that we can heal our bodies and re-connect with our natural environment, inside and out.

Only by disconnecting ourselves from the world of non-stop connectivity can we begin to see how disconnected we have become. And only by reuniting with our true nature, *in nature*, will we see how much of ourselves has gone 'offline'. In connecting with other like-minded individuals, many electro-sensitive people have found the community, compassion, understanding, respect and acceptance that they failed to get in the fast-paced, technologically driven world.

1. Finding our voice

Although our dysfunction is born out of negative subconscious beliefs, belief is not what matters most in healing ourselves and our environment. A strong voice, backed by assertive action, emboldens us and enhances our self-worth. When we hear ourselves speak the deeper truth, our minds and bodies listen, impressed with what we are telling the world and ourselves, in the process. This is what our environment and other people represent for us—a way for us to hear and see ourselves being powerful, compassionate, inspired, eco-aware, creative and everything else we can uniquely be when we give ourselves permission to be autonomous human beings.

Our story must change from one of ill-health, loss and debilitation, to one of renewed health and resilience.

In speaking with a strong voice, we must embrace the deeper truth of who we are and completely let go of the story that has been running our lives. Real as it has been, our story must change from one of ill-health, loss and debilitation, to one of empowered self-healing, positive focus, and renewed health and resilience. When we positively transform our story and the words that shape it, the neuroplasticity of our brains goes to work, creating healthy new neural pathways that reduce our negative expectations and cue the brain to begin restoring balance, which then reduces our anxiety and reactivity, helps to heal any trauma in the limbic brain, and makes us more physically resilient to invasive external forces.

Strengthening our brains

This is not to say that microwave sickness/electro-sensitivity is not real. It most certainly is. However, if we keep telling our brain that the world is not safe, it keeps us in an alarmed, defensive state. In this mode, we become our own worst enemies, living in a state of perpetual fear and battle-readiness that weakens our immune system, kills our hopes and diminishes our capacity for healing. If, however, we affirm that we are strong, resilient and healthy, that we love being in our body, and that we are always safe, we can train our brain to increasingly protect and revitalize us, while doing all we can to live in a natural, low-EMF environment that supports our holistic well-being.

We must also accept responsibility for not having taken responsibility for far too long. This means looking closely at our daily choices, the things we do to either enrich or deplete ourselves and our natural resources, and how we have inadvertently contributed to the radiation-riddled lifestyle that is harming all forms of life and making so many of us ill.

2. Separating ourselves from what separates us

If we are being exposed to radiation that's harming us, our top priority must be to find a safe, healthy place to live. It could be a trailer, a boat, a cabin in the woods or a small single dwelling that we can shield against microwave radiation. Regardless of how challenging that might seem, being absolutely determined to somehow find it is part of the solution and the start of the healing process. When we decide that nothing in the world will stop us from finding a safe place, we will find it. Having faith in our ability to manifest a positive solution may be the first sign we get of what's possible when we start to focus our minds on reclaiming our autonomy. Many of those with electro-sensitivity live in an apartment building and are constantly surrounded by radiation from their neighbours, most of whom typically refuse to turn off WiFi when asked. Continuing to live in this environment of rejection and lack of consideration is not conducive to healing or healthy self-worth (and the same is true in any unhealthy relationship.) Saying *no* to that situation is our first step in saying *yes* to healing ourselves.

If we remain exposed to the electromagnetic radiation that's harming us, it starts to be all that we can see and it can take over our lives. Even if we desperately want to escape, it can distract us from the bigger picture—from the call to empowerment that this disempowering situation is challenging us to embrace. We must disengage so that we can see what has been missing and then engage in a new way, from the inside out. Defining and doing what truly supports, nourishes and enhances us and our planet must be our sole criterion in moving forward.

Finding a low-EMF place to live and/or shielding our living environments gives our bodies a chance to recover. Unless we can prevent ongoing over-stimulation, triggering and stressing of our nervous systems by electromagnetic radiation, we cannot sleep properly, relax, heal or let go of our fear. We must summon the courage, positive intent and, most of all, determination to heal ourselves. We must create a sanctuary for healing as we practise engaging our strong voice, re-writing our story, re-wiring our brains and envisioning a strong comeback into an environment that welcomes, hears and respects us.

Remembering how things really work

When you find a safe spot, away from electromagnetic radiation, and you sit quietly, perhaps unable to do much at all, if you are extremely electro-sensitivity, you may start to hear the frenzy of your mind—all the stories, fears, resentment, anger and frustration of not being able to live your life as you choose. In that stillness, which may feel like an emptiness, you may begin to sense who you really are.

Staying busy and distracted
keeps the truth at bay.

Being marginalized/incapacitated by electro-sensitive represents an opportunity for us to detach from the world and to see it for what it really is: a world of frenzied yet fragmented connectivity, far removed from our true essence. The deeper connection that we yearn for comes from understanding how life really works. When we regain that deeper connection to universal intelligence (which is the same intelligence inside and accessible to us all), we can engage our higher minds to change our external reality, rather than hoping that circumstances will somehow change in our favour. We have been led to believe that change happens outside us and then determines how we feel (which is based on Newton's model of separation), yet the deeper truth is that we, as quantum creators, can—and must—change ourselves inside if we want to take control of our lives and our environment.

What state are you in?

As a human being, what is your most consistent state of being? Is it one of gratitude, contentment or mindful awareness? Or is it anxiety, uncertainty or stress? We are neurologically equipped to change our state of being, which ultimately changes our reality. Instead of allowing the negative memories and experiences of our past to define our expectations of the future, we can invite our future into our present, giving it the context, emotions and qualities that we desire to experience in that unfolding reality.

Embracing a deeper truth

Once we understand that we create the scenarios we call life, and we start to get a sense of how that works, we realize that there is a deeper truth beyond our circumstances. Anyone who challenges or harms us represents an opportunity for us to grow and to take responsibility for what we attract into our lives. It's a chance to weed out our negative programs and replace them with conscious wise choices and proactive engagement. Whether it's a violation of our rights by government agencies or a conflict with a partner, the dynamic is the same. When we get the message and seize the opportunity for greater autonomy, we see things in a very different light. If we take this high road of enlightened self-responsibility, we open the door to true empowerment, which means we regain control over our lives.

A new way of perceiving your aggressors...

See them not as your enemies but as your teachers. Think of them not as an aggressive force but as the resistance you need to work with in order to strengthen your spiritual and emotional muscles. See them not as oppressors but as the impetus that inspires you to reclaim your autonomy. Instead of resenting them, give thanks for what they are showing you and for the wake-up call that we all so clearly need in order to save our selves and our planet from our own dysfunction. Be mindful of their mirroring of our self-destructive behaviours and addictions. Be grateful for the reminder of who you really are and for the fact that no one can keep you stuck in subservience.

See yourself not as the victim of greed or insensitivity, but as the way-shower to those who have lost sight of what it means to be fully human. Be grateful for your infinite capacity for awareness, creativity and growth. Stay conscious of your role in the evolution of our species and your capacity to manifest the life you envision. Trust in the perfection of you, in the power of you, and in your pivotal role as a co-creator. Welcome the clues and the cues leading you towards consciousness and your rightful place on the cosmic stage. Be grateful for your connection to the infinite universal intelligence that infuses our hearts and spirits with the power to transform our planet.

Embrace your destiny.

Answer the call.

It's time to find your way back.

59 Holistic help for the body: what worked for me

Every body is different, with its own unique needs, stressors, constitution, upbringing, wisdom and nutritional requirements. Reclaiming your autonomy and taking back responsibility for yourself means figuring out what works for you—what boundaries to create, choices to make, thoughts to think, foods to eat, people to befriend, exercise to get, and spiritual discipline to embrace. What worked for me may not work for you, and choosing what's best for you enables you to work that all-important 'muscle' of self-determination.

There are many different forms of yoga, for example, and not all of them appeal to everyone. I find kundalini yoga to be the most powerful for me, as it's a very dynamic form with lots of movement, variety and breathwork. Since I spend so much time in my head, this form of yoga puts me back in touch with my body, stilling my mind so that the body can be at peace and I can more readily connect with my own inner guidance. For others, however, hatha yoga or qigong might be best. It's your body and only you can decide.

If you're not used to making certain decisions for yourself, it can take some practice, but there are no wrong choices. Every choice you make will take you on a particular path with particular lessons. If you are open to learning the lessons and embracing whatever gifts present themselves along the way, your evolution will be faster and a lot more fun. Remember: *you* are running the show, even if you're not always conscious of how/why you attract certain things into your life. So there's no point in making yourself wrong for something; just change your mind, choose again and be grateful for having that powerful, uniquely human option.

The most important thing you can do is put yourself first in healthy, practical ways—saying no to unhealthy compromises, following your gut instinct, feeding yourself well, expressing the truth as you see it, maintaining healthy boundaries, and loving yourself just as you are.

Here are some of the things that helped me regain my health and resilience, strengthen my emotional core, and reconnect with my spirituality.

Nutrition and supplements

A healthy diet and the right kind of supplementation can help to counter the many adverse effects of electromagnetic radiation. Since EMR reduces the production of melatonin, causes clumping of red blood cells, affects calcium levels, creates inflammation, weakens the blood–brain barrier, generates free radicals, and generally depletes the body, several specific supplements are needed to target these aspects. (Those I suggest here are for information purposes only, since I am not a medical expert. Check with your doctor, naturopath or healthcare practitioner before taking them—and, of course, do your own due diligence so you can make an informed decision.)

- **Anti-oxidants** help to eliminate the free radicals that cause degeneration and accelerated aging. One particular product—Seanol—made from brown seaweed, is known to cross the blood–brain barrier, thereby providing nutrients and anti-oxidant benefits to the brain. Other anti-oxidants include vitamin C (I usually take buffered vitamin C, in a pure powdered form, as well as quercetin and bioflavonoids, which optimize the body's use of this vitamin), vitamin A, vitamin E and rutin, among others.

- **Anti-inflammatories** help to protect those parts of the body (such as the gut) that can suffer from chronic inflammation. There are many supplements on the market, Theracurmin is a particularly potent and highly bio-available anti-inflammatory derived from turmeric.

- **Melatonin is the body's only built-in free-radical scavenger.** It also regulates sleep, protects against cancer, regulates the immune system and helps protect the gastro-intestinal lining. Insomnia is a common symptom among those who have been affected by EMR, and taking melatonin can help. I have taken large doses (of 10–20mg) when my melatonin levels became severely depleted as a result of chronic EMR exposure.

- **Bio-identical hormones** can be helpful for those whose hormones have become depleted or are out of balance due to chronic stress, aging or degeneration. For women, taking natural progesterone capsules can help with sleep as well as countering any estrogen dominance. But balancing hormones is an art in itself and it requires the input of a skilled and knowledgeable professional who can correctly assess and adjust whatever hormones may be out of balance. Compounding pharmacies may be able to recommend a doctor in your area who can help with this.

- **B complex is needed to counter chronic stress**. This combination of B vitamins supports the nervous system, digestion and many other essential functions. It's important to find a good source of these vitamins—and naturally derived Bs are best of all—so that the body can properly absorb and utilize them. The methylcobalamin form of B12, which targets the nervous system, may also be particularly beneficial for those whose nervous system has been affected.

- **Cleansing and detoxifying supplements** can help you rid the body of accumulated toxins from radiation and other sources. These include chlorella and zeolite—a clay that alkalizes the body and pulls radiation, as well as many other toxins, out of the tissues and cells so that they can be eliminated. Keeping the elimination channels open is therefore important, so that the liberated toxins can be expelled, instead of being re-absorbed back into the tissues.

- **Probiotics and fermented foods boost the good guys in your gut**. The health of the intestinal tract has a huge impact on nutrient absorption, mood, immune function, brain health, and overall well-being. Taking a good probiotic supplement with at least five different strains of healthy bacteria, as well as fermented foods such as sauerkraut and miso, will help to promote the growth of the right kind of bacteria in your gut. It is important to minimize your intake of sugar, since it feeds the 'bad guys' and can cause a proliferation of undesirable bacteria that can undermine your health.

Properly hydrating the body is a fundamental requisite for health that is often overlooked. Dehydration is one of the many effects of chronic EMR exposure, and drinking plenty of pure water throughout the day greatly boosts resilience as well as facilitating regular elimination and ensuring proper electrical conductivity/communication between cells.

Different bodies do well on different diets, and no one diet will work for everyone. While I like the idea of being a vegetarian, it simply doesn't work for my body, no matter how diligently I try to eat this way. I find that a Paleo diet works best for me, as I do well on lots of healthy fats/oils that fuel the brain, as well as lots of vegetables and good-quality animal protein that balances blood sugar and provides sustained energy as well as omega 3s (if it's grass-fed beef/lamb), B12 and lots of other nutrients.

Minimizing my exposure to EMFs

There are several things you can do to reduce the levels of EMFs coming from the wiring and dirty electricity in your home and from your computer and Internet cables. Finding a computer with low EMFs can also make a big difference in your level of daily exposure to electromagnetic radiation.

- **An Ethernet grounding adapter** can be particularly helpful as it greatly reduces the radio-frequency radiation coming through the cables to our computers. (See http://bit.ly/2mzCPie for the adaptor and see http://bit.ly/2Fw10WV for a helpful video on how to set it up, by Jeromy Johnson. More excellent tips on Jeromy's site: http://bit.ly/2ozDPTy.)

- **Shielded Internet cables** further reduce the EMFs coming to and from your computer and, from there, into your body. Cat7 is thought to be the best one to buy. (See, for example, http://amzn.to/2EV8qpR.)

- **A sine wave tamer (or SineTamer)** attached to the electrical panel senses any transient anomalies and mitigates the energy through its internal circuitry to bring back the sine wave form to near-normal flow. Dirty electricity is removed before it enters the home, bringing significant health benefits to occupants and making the power pure for appliances to function normally. I have had many long conversations with Terry Stotyn, who is an expert in this technology, and I'm glad to have this device in our home as it reduced my symptoms within a short time of it being installed.

  "This is the only suppressor that provides this level of protection," Terry tells me, "and our lab in Florida is certified for testing all suppressors manufactured, so we get the opportunity to view all such products on the market." In my research, I have discovered that some even introduce harmonics into the electrical circuitry. SineTamer offers the lowest let-through voltages, Terry tells me, typically bringing the transient activity down to about 1.5% of the original spike levels, as well as filtering radio-frequency and electromagnetic interference from 1kHz to 10MHz. Dr Samuel Milham (in his book, *Dirty Electricity*) states that frequencies from 2kHz to 100kHz are detrimental to human cell structure and are carcinogenic if the body is exposed to them for an extended period of time. (See http://www.cratuscanada.com/ for more info on SineTamers.)

Meditation, stillness and grounding/earthing

Since microwave radiation is known to agitate the nervous system, finding stillness and peace is crucial for those who are electro-sensitive. Meditating daily is one of the most powerful ways to do this as it brings the brain into a more healing state, promotes more restful sleep and gives the body a chance to rest. Peace in the mind creates stillness in the body, and we need both in order to regain our health and vitality.

I find the Six Directions La Chi meditation to be particularly powerful, as if focuses on the body's innate ability to heal itself. See http://bit.ly/2Fcnb6L.

Being in nature is also deeply restorative for mind and body. When we take the time to closely observe nature, we slow down our heart rate and become more present, letting go of the past and future. Grounding by walking barefoot on the earth also generates huge benefits for our health. It reduces the inflammation that so often occurs as a result of us no longer being in close contact with the earth, due to wearing rubber-soled shoes and living in high-rise dwellings. By grounding, we also reconnect with the natural energy that resonates in harmony with our body's electromagnetic fields.

Some people maintain that using grounding mats or other grounding devices in a high-EMF environment will cause those currents to go to ground via your body, which acts as a conductor. However, grounding ourselves in nature, walking barefoot on the earth, away from man-made EMFs, is highly beneficial. For details of the beneficial effects of earthing on inflammation, the immune response, wound healing, and the prevention and treatment of chronic inflammatory and auto-immune diseases, See http://bit.ly/2EVI07u.

Being mindful and positive, and making wise choices

Being aware of our self-talk and ensuring that our thoughts, words and actions are positive and uplifting generates positive outcomes in all areas of life. What we most focus on, in our minds, is what we will attract into our lives.

Our brains and our subconscious minds are our greatest allies in creating the health and the environment that we desire. Both are always listening and will work with whatever raw material we give them, in the form of thoughts, words and actions. We must feed them wisely if we want them to serve our best interests.

I find it particularly effective to listen to my own recorded affirmations. It's relaxing and reassuring to hear myself speaking calmly, confidently and wisely about who I really am and what I'm capable of.

Avoiding unhealthy compromises, having healthy boundaries, making time for self-care and proper nourishment, and being discerning in the company we keep—all serve to keep us emotionally and physically strong. And how we treat ourselves determines how others treat us, so it makes sense to be our own best friend and to treat ourselves well. In the process of doing what's healthy and best for ourselves, we may save lives, heal hearts and make new connections.

Kundalini yoga

As Vancouver-based Kundalini yoga teacher Gloria Latham says, "Wisdom lives in the heart, not your head. The heart guides us to peace, to love and to happiness." And practising yoga every day can take you there, reconnecting you with your heart, your inner wisdom and your soul. This form of yoga has strengthened my emotional core, helped me let go of old patterns and negative emotions, generated a feeling of deep peace, and put me back in touch with my own inner wisdom. It's also a dynamic workout, stimulating all of the body's systems and muscle groups.

Getting myself straightened out

Like many aspects of holistic well-being, the musculoskeletal system is often overlooked in terms of its importance to our overall balance and healthy functioning. The ground-breaking work of postural therapist Pete Egoscue (discussed in chapter 41), who has a unique understanding of the body, provides a vital missing piece of the healing puzzle. His simple exercises and approach will help to get you straightened out and pain-free, usually without the need for invasive surgery or drugs. See www.egoscue.com.

NUCCA (National Upper Cervical Chiropractic Association) is another specialized approach to correcting misalignments. Focusing on re-aligning the atlas (the joint upon which the skull rests), the NUCCA technique can have a profound impact on overall health. When the atlas is out of alignment, the flow of energy and nutrients between the brain and the body is greatly reduced, and all the joints of the body must compensate for the imbalance so that you don't fall over. Migraines, back/neck pain, hip misalignments, having one leg appear to be longer than the other, bone degeneration, and many other conditions can be alleviated when the atlas is adjusted. For me, after the physical trauma of surgery threw my spine out of alignment, this technique proved to be pivotal.

Changing my mind and my reality

Going beyond our usual mental processes and behaviours is crucial to breaking free from limiting patterns and realities. If we neglect our higher spiritual faculties and the phenomenal neuroplasticity of our brains, we deny ourselves a far easier and more powerful pathway to fulfillment.

Working with the principles of neuroplasticity and quantum physics opened up a whole new world of possibilities for me, making me aware of just how much of my brain remains untapped yet available for creating what I want, once I understand how it works. In doing this work, I am reminded of our ongoing ability to tap into universal intelligence, which offers an infinite source of inspiration and support, as well as the quantum field, where all potentialities reside.

The work of Dr Joe Dispenza and the Mastering Alchemy courses offered by Jim Self are just two examples of teachings that can help you access and activate your higher faculties for healing and evolution. See the 'recommended resources' section for more info.

Remembering to play and have fun

Life can seem deadly serious if we are unwell or feeling shaky, lonely, vulnerable or unloved. Movement, laughter and play help us to lighten up and defuse internal stress or anxiety. We need the physical release that comes from getting out of our heads and into our bodies. This is especially true for those who are affected by EMFs, since ongoing stress and worry weaken the immune system and make us more susceptible to depletion and disease.

Vigorous aerobic exercise, laughter with friends, and playing with a child or a dog—all invigorate the body and release feel-good chemicals that enhance our mood and make us feel more positive. Bouncing on a large outdoor trampoline, playing table tennis just for fun (and not keeping score), and finding creative ways to engage (such as playing what I call 'silly Scrabble', which involves making up words and definitions), have been particularly effective ways for me to rest my overly-analytical mind and enjoy myself.

Regularly having fun with friends and loved ones and being creative has helped me to stay focused on what matters most in life. It also keeps my brain engaged in dynamic neural re-wiring so that it brings me more of what I enjoy.

We are highly complex beings yet our most fundamental needs can be simple when we remember what life is all about: loving ourselves, being open to new experiences, having meaningful relationships, allowing the universe and others to support us, living in harmony with our environment, and being all that we can be, in this world of infinite possibilities.

60 Game-changers: playing by the quantum rules

1. **Consciously change your perspective of everything related to EMFs**—and anything else in your world that's not working for you. When you think of EMFs, think: *Elevating My Frequency. Everyone's My Friend! Enjoying My Freedom!* Choose to put a positive spin on whatever has had negative or scary connotations for you in the past. This is not to deny the reality of what's happening out there; it's to reinforce the reality of what's inside you—tremendous power to change your world and start manifesting the life you want. Change your mind and you will change your life.

2. **Find/create a healthy home environment.** Regardless of your circumstances, *know* that you can either move to a better place or modify your existing surroundings to your benefit. Be mindful of any resistance or objections. *I can't move* or *I'm stuck here* is just your negative programming (and fear-driven ego) trying to keep you stuck. It's a reflection of a limited way of thinking and a failure to acknowledge the power you have to attract some unimagined healthy scenario into your life. Yes, you can do this. If you don't, it's not because it's impossible, it's simply because you *believe* it to be impossible. There's a world of difference.

3. **Feed your vision of your ideal future**. Envision your ideal healthy environment and start to focus on that reality. Imagine it, feel it, get excited about it and continually give thanks for it. Believe in it, give it life and make it just as real in your mind than your current reality.

4. **Have faith in yourself and in the universe to co-create something wonderful**. This is crucial to your personal evolution. If you baulk at this step, due to fear or some limiting belief, your efforts are likely to fall short of your expectations and bring mixed results. Having faith in yourself and the universe (which is really the same thing) means you can tap into the infinite possibilities out there in the quantum field, awaiting your instructions and dynamic engagement.

5. **Send positive, health-enhancing messages to your brain and body.** If you are aware of being exposed to radiation and can feel its effects, affirm out loud that you are strong, resilient and robustly healthy. Even if you just anticipate being exposed, do the same thing. Catch yourself in the moment of being triggered, primed for the old way of thinking, defensiveness and/or blame. Take charge of your thinking and take the electrical charge out of it.

6. **Consciously choose how you want to feel** (rather than being a reaction to others or to some external circumstances). Don't let others win by reacting to them in a negative way. Don't give them that power over you. Stay present to the deeper truth of who you are and don't let them win by allowing your own mind to weaken your body/brain through fear or negative projections.

7. **Keep choosing the high road, remembering how things really work.** It's not about letting industry or other wrongdoers off the hook. It's about priming your brain and body to be strong in the face of any perceived threat, while simultaneously elevating your frequency and your capacity to have a positive impact on your environment. Working from the inside out, as well as from the outside in, is the only way that we will turn this situation around.

8. **Don't let yourself down.** Don't give in, don't give up, and don't give out (in Ireland, *giving out* means complaining, which only makes you a victim and a key player in whatever drama surrounds you).

9. **Catch yourself in the instant of self-betrayal.** As soon as you are emotionally triggered and about to go back into a state of fear and anxiety (about EMFs or anything else), say: *STOP! CHANGE! CHOOSE!* Declare the deeper truth and what you consciously want to choose in that moment. *I choose health and resilience. I choose strength and vibrancy. I choose to be well. I choose to elevate my emotions and my frequency. I choose to be stronger than my environment.* Then envision that reality with positive feelings and deep gratitude for it being as good as done.

10. **DO NOT WORRY.** Doing so will only pull you back into the old paradigm of enslavement—to your past, your negative beliefs and your pre-programmed subservience to authority. Fear, doubt and defeat are beneath you, given your creatorship. The only thing you should ever doubt is your negative conditioning. Everything else in you is pure magic.

11. **Stay conscious of being conscious.** You are more consciousness than you are matter or anything else. And consciousness has far more power than matter does, since matter is merely the end result of our mental projections and emotional focus.

12. **Be the change that you want to see.** Make whatever changes in yourself that you want to see reflected back to you in your life, your environment and your relationships. If you want to have more, you must *be* more. If you want something to change, *you* must change.

13. **Bring back respect and send the right message.** Talking on a cell phone while being served by a waiter or at a checkout is disrespectful to that person and reflects low self-worth. By not being present, you are telling them that whoever you are talking to is more important than they are— and that you need to feel important.

14. **Create healthy boundaries.** Don't make or respond to work-related calls or send e-mails on the weekend. We have become impatient and intolerant, expecting things to be done immediately and on our terms. Our boundaries define us, sending out a clear message about what we think about ourselves and how others should treat us. Taking time out, switching off your phone/computer and not making yourself constantly available enhances your self-worth and makes you a more precious 'commodity'. You command respect by having these healthy boundaries, while showing others that you expect the same kind of respect from them.

15. **Stop multi-tasking and be present.** Texts and e-mails may be transmitted almost instantly, but that doesn't mean you must drop whatever you're doing or interrupt a conversation in order to immediately respond to it. Stay focused in the moment, which is where the magic is.

16. **Get whatever emotional and spiritual support you need to become empowered.** Find an enlightened mentor and guide to help you power up. There are many fabulous tools, books and meditations out there (such as those offered by Dr Joe Dispenza and Jim Self[104]) that will help you positively re-program your mind and re-wire your brain. I have no vested interest in recommending these teachers ...other than wanting you to become the amazing creator that you already are, because that helps every one of us.

Conclusion
There's an urgent call for you: do you want to take it?

Microwave sickness/electro-sensitivity is a symptom of what we have lost as human beings—our spiritual connection to the natural world, to universal intelligence, and to our innate creatorship. It represents the last straw in a long line of transgressions against our bodies and our planet. Because so many things in our consumer-driven world (such as our food and medicine) have been de-natured, we have become increasingly disconnected from what is natural and essential for our well-being. Many of us do not know what it feels like to be vibrantly healthy and may not realize just how unhealthy we have become. We see sickness and disease as a normal, inevitable part of life. As more and more gadgets take over our human functions, we are also becoming increasingly de-humanized.

Dealing with electro-sensitivity is all about getting reconnected—with our hearts, with our deeper spiritual selves and our higher faculties, with nature and with each other. It's not just about addressing our symptoms or the harm being caused to us, although we must take care of ourselves like never before. It's about addressing the wider issue of our disempowerment and digging deep, while aiming high, to create the kind of lifestyle and environment that truly serve and nourish us.

While the wireless telecoms industry gears up for a network of electronic interconnectedness that spans the globe, we must get spiritually and collectively connected even faster, activating our full and powerful selves and connecting to the *real* power—not just the external projection of it in the form of our wireless devices. Our hunger for high-tech gadgets reflects not only our deep unmet need for spiritual connection, but also our failure to become fully activated human beings, since we have the potential (once fully conscious and empowered) to do many of the things that our gadgets do.

The body is our medium for processing and generating life, and this is where we must focus if we want to change anything. We do not have to suffer injustices doled out by government or industry. We can take action, from the inside out—co-creating with universal intelligence and serving as curators, willingly and lovingly bringing our bodies and our planet back into balance, with healthy food, wise choices, and conscious self-care. We must treat ourselves the way we want to be treated. We must embody the change we want to see and we must show government and industry what that looks like. *We* set the standard, by virtue of how we treat ourselves, and *we* create the demand—either for more wireless devices, or for technologies, industries and governments that respect us as multi-dimensional beings with hearts, souls and life-saving sensitivity.

Setting a new standard

Reclaiming our personal and environmental health requires a two-pronged approach (described in Chapter 58)—just as our dysfunction evolved along two primary evolutionary paths. Understanding that evolution might help us to retrace our steps back to wholeness and a sense of true belonging.

On the one hand, the negative programming that generated low self-worth, neediness and a sense of powerlessness created in us an insatiable appetite for things to distract us from our pain and compensate for what's missing. The accumulation of more and more gadgets leads to more and more external distraction, which leads to more emotional disconnection, which leads to more reactivity and neediness, which leads to more texting, e-mailing, multi-tasking, over-stimulation and stress, which leads to mental and sensory overload and, ultimately (for those with electro-sensitivity), results in increasing physical, emotional and social isolation. Thus, the very thing we most need—human connection in the form of love and acceptance—is the very thing we end up losing.

On the other hand, surrendering responsibility for self and deferring to others to fix and manage us has created an unhealthy co-dependence and an expectation that things will be taken care of. This results in us having less and less control over our food, health, medicine, politics, industry and environment, which disconnects us from nature and the source of what nourishes and heals us, which further disconnects us from our own healing powers, our need for grounding in the earth and our need for untainted natural resources, which increases our dependence on drugs or other external fixes, which further diminishes our sensitivity to what's healthy for us and the planet, which takes us even further down the rabbit hole of disconnection from our deeper humanity. Once again, our dysfunction has foiled our attempts to make ourselves okay. What we hoped to gain by deferring to authority has resulted in us having almost no authority at all.

Our focus on externalities distracts us from our innate power to create a life of balance, interconnectivity and mutual reward. We cannot conceive of not surviving. Nature has always been there and we expect it to continue, no matter what we throw at it or at ourselves. In essence, we have become addicted to the stress and drama due to our emotional wounds. If we are deeply immersed in our emotional dysfunction, it can be hard to see what is healthy, what is possible or even what it means to be human.

Telling a new story

We must tell a new story that affirms our worthiness and our essential humanity, while engaging our higher faculties. We must also adjust our definitions for what matters most in life. Profit is seen as a monetary gain for one side, rather than a win for all. A thriving economy is considered to be the linchpin of our existence, rather than being the natural outcome of us all thriving together. Sustainability is something that companies think they can buy by paying a tax, rather than something that depends entirely on our collective wise use of shared resources. Governance has come to mean supporting industry, rather than serving and empowering the people that industry is intended to serve. And electro-sensitivity has been ridiculed, rather than being seen as an early-warning system for mankind and a call to embrace our spiritual and emotional selves in developing a sustainable, balanced, mature, respectful way of life.

If our environment is, indeed, the indicator of our evolution and our level of self-mastery, it is clear that we are falling dangerously short of our true potential. Yet our degree of disempowerment represents the flip side of our true capacity to be empowered, autonomous beings. If we embrace the deeper truth of what electro-sensitivity represents, our breakthroughs will be proportionate to how helpless and hopeless many of us have felt. As electro-sensitive individuals, our challenge is therefore not to somehow survive, but to be the lamplighters of a new way of living that integrates our essential humanity, creativity and brainpower with a passion for human betterment, the engagement of our spiritual faculties and a profound respect for our natural world.

It's not the voice of reason but the voice of pure consciousness that must drown out all the other voices competing for supremacy in your mind. Unconscious, reactive living—and conscious, proactive living—brings more of the same. It's just a matter of where we choose to put our focus.

The future is created in this moment. Will we continue to feed the same old story? Or will we consciously feed a vision of vibrant human health and a pristine environment?

The choice is ours.

Afterword by Lewis Evans
(*The Husband*)

Olga asked me to share some thoughts about my experience with her electro-sensitivity and the impact it has had on me.

First, let me tell you, I am not electro-sensitive and I do not feel electromagnetic radiation. It has therefore been challenging for me to understand what Olga feels and how much impact it has had on her, especially when she first discovered her sensitivity. I feel that I should have known, as I was responsible for designing, developing and commercializing one of the very first products intended to protect people from the radiation emitted by mobile phones, back in the 1990s.

So, that's the first emotion I felt: guilt. I was guilty of not realizing that she was being affected. I was guilty of wanting to continue, undisturbed, with my cell phone, wireless computer connection and all the 'convenient' gadgets that I could lay my hands on. After all, that's the way the world works now, isn't it? All business is shifting towards wireless connectivity at an accelerating rate, and you must use wireless devices if you want to be *cool* and *professional*.

And I felt guilty that I was not, in my heart, putting Olga's health first. It was so damned inconvenient to adjust my life in order for things to work for her, and some part of me, in the early days, thought that she must me making a mountain out of a molehill.

But I am an extremely fortunate man, in that I have an incredible relationship with my wife. I have a lot of respect for her, as well. She is intelligent, witty, heartfelt, has huge integrity, is wise and is fun to be with. She's the only person I know who interviewed a parking meter, a peanut, a toilet and lots of other inanimate objects—with wildly enlightening results.

My love for her runs deeper than I could ever have imagined. Trusting that and trusting her, I found myself gradually ditching the guilt in place of affirmative, supportive action. And, as Olga kept reminding me, I shouldn't feel guilty about giving up the guilt.

It hasn't been a straightforward, linear journey. Even now, I occasionally lapse into feeling petty resentments, quiet annoyance at having to accommodate her sensitivity, and other unhelpful, selfish emotions, which I then admonish myself for feeling …which doesn't help, either!

Having said that, being married to someone with electro-sensitivity has as many blessings as it has inconveniences and challenges. It just depends on your point of view and how you choose to deal with it. I know of others with an electro-sensitive partner but who are not electro-sensitive themselves. If you are one of them, I am sure you can relate to what follows here, and I hope that it's of value to you on your journey with your partner.

I feel I have grown in many ways, since we confirmed electromagnetic radiation as the true cause of Olga's health problems. It wasn't the kind of growth I was looking for, however. I had been looking for economic growth, having spent what I thought was sufficient time and energy on personal growth, so that we could look forward to a nice, financially secure future. That, I told myself, was why I had to be completely up to date with all the latest technology.

But the growth I experienced was more of a 'human' growth. It challenged my values, forced me to confront my sense of self and demanded that I shape up. It was as if life was saying to me, "Okay, let's see what you're really made of. We're going to push all your buttons, mess with your head, strip away all your BS and then see what happens!"

The process involved five key stages that sometimes overlap and sometimes come back for more, just when I think I've resolved them. I have listed them here, with a few examples of the many experiences I have had on this journey.

1. Anger

First, there were the doctors and healthcare practitioners who knew nothing about electro-sensitivity. While some were helpful in relieving some symptoms, Olga usually knew a lot more about her condition than they did. Many were condescending and had a narrow expertise or knowledge that they implemented by rote, without understanding the bigger picture. I can remember one particularly arrogant private doctor in Vancouver. He charged an exorbitant fee for his time, much of which he spent blowing his own trumpet and telling Olga how much he enjoyed his job. This was followed by him imparting particularly useless advice, which failed to address the issue of electro-sensitivity. Some doctors just don't like being told that the patient knows better than they do.

Then there were the suppliers and service-providers—telecoms, electric power, politicians and the justice system—who are technically there to either provide a service or represent citizens and address their concerns, but who operate like some sort of mafia driven by profit.

Most of all, I was angry about the general lack of compassion and humanity. Olga received no assistance or accommodation from the so-called authorities, was dismissed by service-providers, and was unable to assert her legal and human rights due to the lack of enforcement by those who have a duty to uphold them.

2. Frustration

I just wanted my life to continue without all this fuss. I didn't want cables trailing all over the house so we could isolate some rooms from high electrical fields or dirty electricity. I wanted to be able to use my cell phone occasionally because I had given my number out to so many people. After spending weeks looking for a new place to live, the last thing I wanted to hear was that it was problematic, and that I had to shield two entire sides of the house and find all sorts of ways to reduce the harmful fields.

And it was frustrating that our social life was so greatly affected. Olga could not go shopping or socialize much, and we could rarely visit friends for dinner. It was usually too complicated to arrange a safe electrical environment, as people had no understanding of what was required for Olga to be able to relax and enjoy herself and it often felt too awkward to ask them to change things. I either had to go on my own or not at all. Olga always encouraged me to go. It's fortunate that she is quite happy being on her own, but it's frustrating because this was not her choice. I used to enjoy being with her among friends. Just watching her interacting with others is a source of joy for me.

There have been so many frustrations, and I am still coming to terms with some of them. Sometimes I have to catch myself so I don't overreact when they kick in. Many are seemingly trivial, like being reminded every night to turn off a particular and seemingly harmless electric circuit breaker. Of course, it's important to turn off the breaker and I should be thankful for the reminder. But it's what that reminder represents and the long story and heavy baggage behind it, as well as my self-recriminations for my own insensitivity, which inflate its importance. I am therefore having to learn to stand back, take the sting out of all the frustrations and deal with them more maturely. They are simply not worth giving airtime to, and Olga's health is far more important than what they represent.

3. Sorrow

I feel an overwhelming sadness, at times, that Olga's life has become so constricted. She is naturally vivacious. I have never laughed as much with anyone as I have with Olga. As I said, she is witty and wise, and she has a brilliant brain. We have, in the past, enjoyed lots of travel to far-flung places on wonderful holidays. At the time of writing, she can't take a flight anywhere because airplanes now have WiFi and many cities have blanket WiFi coverage.

More than that, though, over the years since her surgery, Olga has rarely been her usual energetic self, due to the cumulative affects of electromagnetic radiation. Whether it is faulty electric wiring in a house, the fields emanating from her computer as she writes, neurological issues due to the surgery to remove her acoustic neuroma, or subsequent damage brought on by consequential factors, she has struggled much of the time.

That we can, as a society, ignore, malign and obstruct the implementation of healthy solutions to the environmental problems that she and so many others face, is sad indeed, and it doesn't bode well for our future. I have always seen Olga as the 'canary in the coal mine', flagging dangers that we all face and are being affected by, whether we are aware of them or not. In my opinion, all electro-sensitive individuals should be thanked for bringing these dangers to our attention at their own expense, both health-wise and financially.

4. Acceptance

As John Lennon famously said, "Life is what happens to you when you're busy making other plans". In our case, life has taken so many unexpected twists and turns that planning has all but been abandoned! Although we still have a strong vision of a wonderful future, I have learned to accept a semi-nomadic lifestyle, with constant uncertainties around where we will live next and how I am going to make a living. On that score, I am fortunate to have wide-ranging skills and experience that I can apply in different situations, but there is always a learning curve when you arrive in a new community. At the time of writing, we are living in the village of Horsefly, BC, in Canada, and it has thus far been a wholly refreshing experience. Here, we have been welcomed as part of a wonderful community, and I now have more friends than I ever had living in any city.

When I think back to how I saw my life panning out from the perspective of a university student, I can only laugh. It has been so much richer since I met Olga in Switzerland than I could ever have imagined. Having survived these recent years with all their stresses and uncertainties, I am beginning to trust that we are being looked after. I no longer fret over what I cannot do, the things I may not achieve and the money I may not make. Acceptance of the current situation and gratitude for all that I have is replacing those negative projections and, ironically, this new state of equilibrium makes me feel that much more is possible for us and that we don't have to concern ourselves with the details.

5. Admiration

I have never admired anyone in my life as much as I admire Olga. You may say I am biased. If so, you can EMF off! I have been privileged to be with her through all her struggles—and I have had a ringside seat, so I see everything! I am in awe of how diligently she researches every possible avenue to resolve her health problems and how she takes on and exposes the corruption, stupidity and blindness of institutions, companies and authorities that are often in complete dereliction of their moral and legal responsibilities. To be the recipient of her love and support when I am fussing over my own relatively minor problems is truly inspiring and somewhat humbling. And she has supported many other electro-sensitive individuals in practical ways. All of this, while she was feeling debilitated, ill and sleep-deprived. When most people would have taken sick leave, she has been a fighter, a seeker and a problem-solver for herself and others.

In recent months, she has emerged from a sense of hopelessness to one of 'robust possibilities'. I feel a stronger Olga emerging, and that energizes me, as well. The work she has been doing on herself has changed her attitude to her situation and has opened up new realms of healing and possibilities. I, too, have changed as we have explored these dimensions together. Despite once believing that our options were becoming more limited, I now have an expanded sense of what's possible and am grateful for all that I have learned.

I cannot wait to see what happens next!

—Lewis Evans
January 2018

Appendix 1: Sources of man-made electromagnetic radiation in our environment

1. Alternating current (AC) electrical fields

Wherever there is electricity, you will have electric and magnetic fields. Termed *power frequency*, these fields are classified as extremely low frequency (ELF) fields because they represent frequencies from zero to 3000Hz. In North America, the power line frequency is 60Hz. These fields radiate out from sources and cause adverse biological effects in living things. Man-made electrical fields are everywhere in our electrified societies. Electrical fields are easily attenuated by grounded and conductive materials and objects, such as trees, buildings and building materials, especially brick, cement board, concrete and various specialty materials that can be used in dwellings for shielding purposes. Electrical field strength is determined by voltage. The higher the voltage or electrical pressure and the shorter the distance to the sources, the stronger and more harmful the fields.

Lamps and appliances with two-wire cords are one of the most significant sources of electrical fields in a home. Even if not turned on, they still emit strong fields while plugged in. Have a professional rewire these with appliances with specialized grounded, shielded cords to reduce these electrical fields.

Before the early 1990s, electric fields were regarded by most EMF-aware health professionals as benign. Subsequent studies showing harm, and activism by scientists not beholden to military/industry interests, gave credence to electrical fields as a serious threat to public health.

In North America, AC power lines, equipment, building wiring and all things electrical expose us to 60Hz energy, which is measurable inside our bodies at this same frequency. They cause undesirable currents to flow inside us that are billions of times stronger than the micro-currents in our own body's electrical system. These currents are a continual presence in all wired structures, unless specially wired and shielded to produce low-EMF conditions (as specified, for instance, by the Institute of Building Biology and Sustainability [IBN, Germany], which recommends levels of less than 1V/m in sleeping areas). They are attracted to the ground and to our bodies, which act as antennae. Many scientists conclude that this is why electrical fields have an association with disorders of the central nervous system.

A 'healthy home' requires minimizing all EMR from areas where most time is spent, the most significant being sleep areas. A low-EMF design mandates that all AC wiring be shielded, metal-clad or enclosed within an electrical conduit and that all electrical boxes be metal. Plastic-coated electrical wiring (Loomex, in Canada; Romex, in the USA), as used in virtually all houses, affords no protective shielding against electric fields. Protecting sleep areas from this harmful contamination is the main priority because we are up to 100 times more vulnerable to stressors during sleep. EMR is known to disrupt melatonin production. There should be no energized wiring, devices etc within 3 metres of sleep areas.

2. Magnetic fields (AC, ELF)

Any device, appliance or power line will produce an alternating current magnetic field. The intensity or strength of the field is directly related to the power consumption involved. In homes and offices, this field generally remains close to its source (up to 2 metres) but it can extend to over 200 metres, as in the case of high-voltage power lines. Power panels and meters (both digital and analog types) and utility service wiring are the most harmful sources of magnetic fields in a home. (Smart meters placed on dwellings require both extremely low frequency (ELF) and radio-frequency shielding.) It is advisable to locate work, leisure and, most importantly, sleep areas well away from panels and related electrical wiring and equipment. Additionally, homes have many appliances emitting levels of up to hundreds of milligauss, which are known to create adverse health effects.

Other sources to be avoided are electrically adjusted beds, electrically heated floors and ceilings, bathtubs and hot tubs with motorized massage jets (unless motors are rewired to be 2–3 metres from the unit), infrared saunas, fluorescent lights, lamps with ballasts (such as compact fluorescent light (CFL) bulbs), clock radios, electric blankets and pads, hairdryers, electronic massagers and far infrared heating pads. Electric cars emit high fields, which manufacturers could render far safer with inexpensive shielding. Other high-current household items include kitchen appliances, electric heaters, electric power tools and transformers.

Another common source of magnetic fields is poor wiring, which poses increased fire and shock risks, as well as health risks from the elevated field that extends far from the wall. The resulting unbalanced currents contaminate a home and promote health disorders. These wiring/grounding flaws can only be detected with skilled use of magnetic field meters and are rarely identified by electricians or electrical inspectors—unless, as is the practice in many European Union jurisdictions, they test the integrity of the wiring using a magnetic field meter. At least 15% of North American housing stock has wiring/grounding-related magnetic fields caused by wiring errors.

Proximity to power lines and equipment, grounding to municipal water piping, corroded wiring, and failure to disconnect neutral bus ground connections in secondary power panels are also sources of magnetic fields in homes.

Magnetic fields are difficult to block by shielding, as they permeate most materials, including the human body. Shielding is expensive and usually somewhat disappointing. Only certain metal alloys such as Mu-metal, G-iron Flex or low-carbon steel sheeting and, to a lesser degree, aluminum, can be useful when applied.

Magnetic fields penetrate the body and tend to afflict the organs and endocrine system. At low exposure levels, there are increased risks of adverse pregnancy outcomes, and of diseases/conditions such as childhood leukemia, cancer, tumours, migraines, pain, depression, heart disease, increased suicides and sleep disorders, as well as disorders of the hormone, nervous, reproductive and cardiovascular systems.

3. Radio-frequency radiation, radio-frequency/microwave radiation, high-frequency, non-ionizing electromagnetic radiation (also referred to as wireless radiation)

Radio-frequency (RF) radiation is the core component of our wireless communication infrastructure, as well as being central to extensive military warfare applications. RF and microwave-frequency waves can convey information from one place to another through the air, as they do via numerous wireless devices/systems, such as cordless phones, cell phones, cell towers, smart meters, microwave ovens, WiFi, WLAN, tablets, iPads and the myriad other sources. They are also used in radio and TV broadcasts, radar, satellite navigation and homeland security, among many other things. These high-energy waveforms are more intense, further reaching and more harmful than low-power frequency radiation. Radio frequency extends from 3kHz (3,000Hz) to 3GHz (300 billion hertz). Microwaves are a sub-category of RF, in the range of 300MHz to 300GHz, which is the range used in modern communications.

For most of Earth's history, the electromagnetic spectrum consisted mainly of natural, direct current (DC) electromagnetic phenomena such as visible light, lightning, radiation from space, and the magnetic field of the Earth. Before the late 1920s, when radio became widespread, Earth was a fundamentally different planet. Today and increasingly into the future, every conceivable commercial, military and recreational use of the electromagnetic spectrum is being exploited, with virtually no protective measures taken and with minimal consideration by governments, health authorities and an unwitting public for the proven adverse biological effects of this electro-pollution.

Electromagnetic high-frequency radiation, including all things wireless, consist of electric and magnetic waves that are coupled. They are no longer separate entities. Alternating current (AC) electric and magnetic fields continually recreate each other at the speed of light to infinity. The shorter the wavelength, the higher the frequency and the more biologically active the radiation becomes, the higher its potential for harm.

AC electric and magnetic fields become airborne from about 3kHz to 300GHz. Electric and magnetic fields in the radio-frequency/microwave range are measured together as power density, and also in volts per meter. Each RF signal consists of a high frequency 'carrier signal' and a second 'modulated' signal that carries the voice, images and computer data, at ELF frequencies similar to those of brain waves and electricity, and very close to the energy patterns of the Earth and our bodies. Accordingly, these information-carrying waves readily interact with and disrupt various body and brain functions. Now, with 5G technology, the telecoms industry is poised to increase use of the highest and most penetrating gigahertz range.

Our modern societies are fast becoming entirely wireless. These increasing RF sources overpower the subtle signals of the natural background from space and Earth—the very conditions that created every life form. No place on the planet will remain untouched by man-made radiation. The ubiquitous irradiation of citizenry (with consideration only of engineering efficacy) continues unabated, spurred on by the demands of a misinformed public for faster download speeds. New satellite systems will soon add to existing space-based transmitters to saturate the planet with high-powered pulsed digital microwaves, as will irradiating balloons suspended at high altitudes to provide high-speed Internet services to rural regions.

4. Static electrical fields

These fields result from the build-up of airborne electricity around materials charged with static electricity. High levels can create sparks, which can cause explosions around various volatile chemicals. For healthy living/working conditions, it is best to use materials that do not retain static charge and that discharge efficiently. Adverse air-quality problems result from the use of synthetic materials holding static charges in buildings. Forced-air heating can also cause a build-up of positively charged air, aggravating adverse physical symptoms. Static electricity is known to cause stress and tension in people and animals, and it increases dramatically when air humidity falls below 40%. Symptoms include pressure in the head area, fatigue, low blood pressure, respiratory difficulties and general loss of vitality.

5. Static magnetic fields

The Earth's magnetic field is an indispensable aspect of the biology of every living thing, and an essential navigational tool for all species. Unlike DC magnetic fields, static magnetic fields penetrate bodies, where they cause undesirable electrical fields to be generated within body tissue.

Metals near the body act as antennae/amplifiers that increase, re-radiate and reflect ambient high-frequency radio-frequency/microwave electromagnetic radiation into the body. The presence of metals near or under the body is quite harmful during sleep, due to the RF amplification effects, and because magnetized metals (steel, nickel etc) interfere with the natural geomagnetic field of the Earth, upon which all life depends for orientation. Beds, particularly, should be free of metals, given these factors. It is important to have no sudden variations in the natural geomagnetic field in sleeping areas. Adverse health effects can be aggravated by coil and spring mattresses, metal bed frames, metal artifacts under beds, and metallic furniture (such as office chairs and filing cabinets), as well as from building components such as metal beams, and rebar.

6. Micro surges (dirty electricity/harmonic pollution)

Dirty electricity, also referred to as electromagnetic interference (EMI), is electrical energy or electric power that has been corrupted and distorted by the use of modern appliances. These high-frequency harmonic distortions travel along wiring, from outside and inside sources. They degrade electrical equipment, which is designed only for 'clean' (60Hz) electricity, and escape from power lines and electrical wiring and equipment, becoming radio-frequency fields that cause harm to living things. Inside sources include: switch-mode power supplies (SMPS), transformers and chargers that convert supplied power into lower/higher voltages and AC into the DC power used by electronics, such as TVs, computers, sound systems, office equipment, low-energy lighting, including all lights with ballasts (especially the hazardous compact fluorescent light (CFL) bulbs), and many models of LED bulbs, dimmer switches and other sophisticated electronics. They greatly increase power bills by wasting energy. They are classed as low-frequency electromagnetic fields, generally in the ELF and VLF range (0 to 30,000Hz).

Solutions include avoiding excess emitters, such as lighting that uses 'non-line voltage' (voltage that is chopped up to power lower energy needs), keeping distance from known sources and using switched power bars (turned off when devices are not in use). A more costly way of reducing internally and externally generated dirty electricity involves installing specialized equipment at the panel to trap and rid the electrical system of harmonic pollution, thus correcting power quality, reducing power bills and protecting occupants' health.

A note about body voltage

Airborne AC electrical fields are always seeking ground. Our bodies are better conductors than air, and they serve as conduits for these active fields. Testing one's body voltage, measured in millivolts (mV), can be a valuable way of identifying the AC voltage present inside a human body in a particular location. It reflects the presence and intensity of AC electrical fields. These tests, carried out with a body voltage meter, are used mainly to identify specific circuits that contaminate sleeping areas, so that remediation measures, such as selective re-wiring, moving beds or using 'demand switches' can be implemented. These automatic switches serve to eliminate electrical fields when power is not required (such as at night) by turning off offending circuits. The ideal body voltage recommended by the Institute of Building Biology and Sustainability is 10 millivolts (mV).

NB: It is beyond the scope of this book to cover all forms of electromagnetic radiation in our environment, but there are two other forms that you might wish to research.

Ionizing radiation is the most lethal form of electromagnetic radiation and it is classified as a known carcinogen at any exposure level. People are exposed to low levels of natural sources of ionizing radiation, such as in soil, water and vegetation, as well as from man-made sources, such as x-rays and medical devices.

While lower-frequency radiation such as ELF (as in electricity) sources and radio-frequency sources induce unwarranted current flows in bodies, as one mechanism of harm, the much more intense ionizing radiation is far more dangerous and damages our DNA more quickly and effectively than its lower energy counterparts. Earth is constantly bombarded by ionizing cosmic radiation, most of which is blocked by Earth's magnetic field and ozone layer.

Radon, a sub-category of ionizing radiation, is a naturally occurring, odourless, colourless radioactive soil gas from the decay of uranium. It is ubiquitous and relatively harmless in outdoor air, but potentially lethal when concentrated in indoor air. Levels vary widely in different geographical locations. This worldwide problem exists where radon seeps into buildings and accumulates, especially where inadequate ventilation exists. It is the leading cause of lung cancer in non-smokers, killing over 20,000, both in the USA and Canada. The EPA recommends radon testing in all homes and buildings whether in high-radon zones or not. There is no known safe level.

Information provided by Chris Anderson, of Electro Smog Solutions, who has over two decades of experience in assessing and minimizing electromagnetic radiation in homes and businesses.

Recommended resources

Recommended websites relating to EMFs, EHS and EMR

On the website of *Microwave News*, there is an excellent directory of EMF/EMR sites around the world. See http://microwavenews.com/www.html.

See also:

- Practical steps for restoring social justice and accountability—InPower Movement: https://InPowerMovement.com/
- Physicians for Safe Technology: https://mdsafetech.org/
- Living with EHS: http://www.weepinitiative.org/livingwithEHS.html
- Conventions, commissions and legal/practical advice re EHS: http://www.electrosensitivity.co/disability-and-access-in-practice.html
- For coverage of the science, policies, facts and resources relating to EMFs, see the Environmental Health Trust, which also produces an excellent newsletter and provides kits for individuals to use in taking action in their communities: https://ehtrust.org/.
- For informative newsletters and other EMF/EMR-related content: http://www.es-uk.info/
- For more information on autism: http://www.marthaherbert.org/
- For tips on reducing EMFs from your computer and Internet cables: https://www.emfanalysis.com/low-emf-computing/
- For cancer research/statistics and other EMF-related info: http://www.wi-cancer.info
- Valuable information and resources from Dr William Rea's Environmental Health Centre–Dallas, which focuses on the relationship of health and disease to environmental factors: https://www.ehcd.com
- A global forum for healing through intention: http://theintentionexperiment.com/
- Sites covering the impact of EMFs/EMR in South Africa and beyond: http://www.emfsa.co.za; http://www.emrsa.co.za; and http://www.emrrfsa.org

- Children in Cape Town singing a song opposing a cell tower in the grounds of a church that houses a crèche: https://www.youtube.com/watch?v=yd1aSav9BVU.
- TV news coverage of people with EHS in South Africa: http://bit.ly/2GMwk3p.
- Wisdom, solutions and practical guidance from Jolie Jones: www.jolietalks.com

Recommended further reading

Books by Dr Joe Dispenza:

- *Breaking the Habit of Being Yourself*
- *Evolve Your Brain—the science of changing your mind*
- *You Are the Placebo—making your mind matter*
- *Becoming Supernatural—how common people are doing the uncommon*

Books by Pete Egoscue:

- *Pain Free—a revolutionary method for stopping chronic pain*
- *Pain Free Living*
- *Pain Free at your PC*

Books by Dr Norman Doidge:

- *The Brain that Changes Itself*
- *The Brain's Way of Healing—remarkable discoveries and recoveries from the frontiers of neuroplasticity*

The Invisible Rainbow: A History of Electricity and Life, by Arthur Firstenberg (http://www.cellphonetaskforce.org/buy-the-invisible-rainbow/)

The Quantum Doctor, by Amit Goswami

Living Safely with Electromagnetic Radiation, by Jim Waugh. See http://www.emfsafehome.com.

The Rebirth of Nature, by Rupert Sheldrake.

The Intention Experiment: Using your thoughts to change your life and the world, by Lynne McTaggart

Light that Heals, by Donna Fisher

Dirty Electricity —Electrification and the Diseases of Civilization, by Dr Samuel Milham

Earthing—The Most Important Health Discovery Ever?, by Clinton Ober, Dr Stephen Sinatra, MD and Martin Zucker. See also: https://www.youtube.com/watch?v=8KxsaZxXEZ0.

Videos/documentaries on EMFs/EHS/EMR

- *Take Back Your Power* 2017: https://vimeo.com/227169236/ed84a782a8

- *Generation Zapped*: https://generationzapped.com/

- Harmful effects of screen time: https://www.youtube.com/watch?v=QGZV-FZ1ggY

- How we are killing ourselves—wireless radiation: http://www.odwyerpr.com/story/public/6751/2016-04-20/israel-wi-fi-breakthroughs-tv-documentary-school-ban.html.

- Breaking bad medicine, by Dr Kelly Brogan: https://www.youtube.com/watch?v=cbsoU7PFBU4.

Acknowledgements

In dealing with the effects of the electromagnetic radiation in our environment, I have experienced some daunting challenges, learned many lessons, made unexpected breakthroughs, and gained new friends. There are many phenomenal people I wish to thank for having joined me on this journey and for enriching my life. In the generous sharing of information, wisdom and life experiences, we have become a community, collaborating and contributing for the sake of our planet.

I am deeply grateful to my husband, Lewis Evans, who is my hero, my steady, loving companion, my biggest fan and my partner in all things. Without him, this book—and our efforts to create a healthier home—would not have been possible.

Chloe Sheean brings new meaning to the term *sister* and never ceases to amaze me with her capacity for positivity, love, encouragement, insights, support and creative shopping for sensitive siblings.

My profound thanks to Denise Rowland for her invaluable insights, editorial assistance, wisdom, humour, caring and friendship. She has helped immeasurably in the writing of this book and in sharing our vision of the future. She has also become a powerful activist and spokesperson on EMR, working tirelessly on behalf of the disadvantaged Cape Town communities being harmed by cell towers in their neighbourhoods.

My sincere thanks also to Karl Muller, who is an ongoing source of inspiration, encyclopedic knowledge, insights and support.

Sarah Benson has been a solid, supportive friend, a source of wry good humour and spiritual insights, and an inspiration to others with her own powerful writing and creative ideas for raising public awareness about EMFs.

Marcus and Benita Schluschen were the first responders—and our first friends—when we moved to Vancouver Island to pursue a healthier, low-EMF lifestyle. They have added significantly to my awareness of the science on EMR and have consistently offered their generous feedback and support.

Lucy Sanford has been a mentor, teacher and true life-saver, embodying the genuine caring, profound self-awareness, and respect for the body's own wisdom that are so often missing from mainstream medicine. She is living proof of the power of the mind to heal the body and overcome even the most daunting odds.

Heartfelt thanks to Maria Vlasopoulos for her deep compassion, healing hands and unsurpassed intuitive bodywork, which greatly enhanced my post-op recovery and helped to offset the effects of EMR.

I would like to thank Christine Zipps for her valuable editorial feedback, support, friendship and dedication to inspiring meaningful action and change.

There are many others who have enhanced my knowledge of electro-sensitivity, offered practical suggestions for minimizing my EMF exposure, and/or provided meaningful support. These include, but are not limited to: Dr Erica Mallery-Blythe, Josh del Sol, Prof. Trevor Marshall, Sarah Dacre, Janis Hoffmann, Sharon Noble, Melissa Chalmers, Kate Kheel, Jolie Jones, Jeromy Johnson, Helène Vadeboncoeur, Dr William Rowland, Anton Fernhout, Norm Ryder, Ed Friedman, Chris Anderson, Olga Aguinaga, and Dave and Wilma Miles.

Finally, I would like to thank the community of Horsefly, in British Columbia, Canada, which has welcomed and supported us in ways that redefine the concept of community. I am particularly grateful to Michelle Wong and Victor Khong, who warmly extended their friendship, shared their extensive knowledge of EMFs, organized fantastic fitness classes, and helped us find a home. And to Pamela, a huge thank-you for the gift of a warm and safe haven throughout the long Cariboo winter, complete with Jake, a super-smart canine who reminds us to play, enjoy nature, and always make time for heartfelt connections.

Notes

1   See http://bit.ly/2ESbi2C.

2   See Dr Bradford S. Weeks, on the coming brain cancer epidemic: http://bit.ly/2ESEaIb.

3   See www.emf-portal.org; https://www.emfanalysis.com/research/; and https://ehtrust.org/science/research-industry-influence-emfs/.

4   *Glow Kids: How Screen Addiction Is Hijacking Our Kids and How to Break the Trance*; http://nyp.st/2ESvFNd.

5   See http://bit.ly/2ESvOAf.

6   The book ends up being a phenomenal geo-political thriller that takes us both by surprise. See http://hominine.info.

7   See https://lewisevans.net/art/.

8   See http://bit.ly/2ETODCW

9   See box on the symptoms of EHS.

10   See http://dailym.ai/2EQlHvO and http://bit.ly/2ERN34J.

11   Diagnosis and management of electromagnetic hypersensitivity (EHS): rapid overview for a mixed audience—a highly informative presentation by Dr Erica Mallery-Blythe at the British Society of Ecological Medicine convention in March 2014 (see https://vimeo.com/100623585).

12   See the excellent work of Dr Andrew Goldsworthy, who explains in detail the biological effects of weak electromagnetic fields: http://bit.ly/2ESF0Vl.

13   Ibid. See also Pall, M. L. (2014). Microwave electromagnetic fields act by activating voltage-gated calcium channels: why the current international safety standards do not predict biological hazard. *Recent Res. Devel. Mol. Cell. Biol.* (7) (available at: http://bit.ly/2ESwIfS).

14   See http://goo.gl/RCiYLa.

15   In 2014, monitors at the Russian Space Observing System showed a sudden spike in activity to around 8.5Hz. Since then, they have recorded days where the Schumann resonance accelerated as fast as 16.5Hz. At first, they thought their equipment was malfunctioning, but the data turned out to be accurate. Everyone was asking what was causing this intermittent spiking activity. Is the

Earth's frequency speeding up? Since the Schumann frequency is said to be in tune with the human brain's alpha and theta states, this acceleration may be why it often feels as if time has sped up and events and changes in our life are happening more rapidly. These emerging resonances are naturally correlated to human brainwave activity, which means that we are changing. See http://bit.ly/2nK0O12.

16   See http://bit.ly/2EV2tVP.

17   See http://www.emfsafehome.com.

18   See http://bit.ly/2ET2WYw among many other sources available online.

19   See https://www.emf-portal.org.

20   The device utilized 'sputter coating' and stealth technology similar to what is used on bombers to hide them from radar and inside the phones to protect components from each other. Lewis had adapted the technology to protect cell-phone users from the radiation hitting their ear—the most vulnerable part of the skull.

21   See http://bit.ly/2EROn7I.

22   *The Alphabet of Powerful Existence—an A–Z guide to well-being, wisdom and worthiness*, 2013. See https://olgasheean.com/the-alphabet-of-powerful-existence/.

23   See https://olgasheean.com/a-talk-on-the-wild-side/.

24   Free download available here: https://olgasheean.com/no-safe-place/.

25   See http://bit.ly/1svnHmQ for more compelling evidence to the contrary.

26   See, for example, http://bit.ly/1RNGwe0.

27   See http://bit.ly/2ESB8Du.

28   See the article by Dr Christine Aschermann in *Umwelt-Medizin-Gesellschaft* (UMG 2010, 3).

29   Dr Andrew Goldsworthy has produced compelling, comprehensive accounts of the multiple effects of EMFs, referencing over 70 scientific studies), the dangers of electromagnetic smog, and why the body is affected the way it is (see http://bit.ly/1PlASJZ; http://bit.ly/28ltGL9; and http://bit.ly/1taEDi3).

30   See Henshaw, DL and Reiter, RJ (2005). Do magnetic fields cause increased risk of childhood leukemia via melatonin disruption? *Bioelectromagnetics Supplement 7*: S86–S97.

31   See Beason and Semm, 2002; Krey and Dolmetsch, 2007, Volkow et al, 2011.

32 From the International EMF Scientist Appeal, which urgently calls upon the United Nations and its sub-organizations, WHO and UNEP, and all UN Member States, for greater health protection on EMF exposure. See http://www.emfscientist.org and http://goo.gl/sLi7Uu.

33 The 2012 *BioInitiative Report* was prepared by 29 authors (including 10 MDs, 21 PhDs, 3 MsCs, MAs or MPHs) from 10 countries (Austria, Canada, Denmark, Greece, India, Italy, Russia, the Slovac Republic, Sweden and the USA). Among the authors is the Chair of the Russian National Committee on Non-Ionizing Radiation, and a Senior Advisor to the European Environmental Agency.

34 Dr Dietrich Klinghardt, MD, PhD, is Founder of the Klinghardt Academy (USA), the American Academy of Neural Therapy, Medical Director of the Institute of Neurobiology, and lead clinician at the Sophia Health Institute (Washington State). He is also Founder and Chairman of the Institute for Neurobiology (in Germany & Switzerland). See https://youtu.be/PktaaxPl7RI and http://www.klinghardtacademy.com/.

35 See https://youtu.be/PktaaxPl7RI and http://www.klinghardtacademy.com/.

36 See http://bit.ly/2ESderU.

37 See http://goo.gl/RCiYLa.

38 See https://youtu.be/PktaaxPl7RI.

39 See also the excellent work of pediatric neurologist and brain development researcher, Dr Martha Herbert: http://www.marthaherbert.org/.

40 Dr Herbert is a paediatric neurologist and neuroscientist at Harvard Medical School and on staff at Massachusetts General Hospital. Board-Certified in Neurology, she specializes in Child Neurology and Neuro-developmental Disorders.

41 See http://bit.ly/1JXLfnr.

42 See https://buildingbiology.com/.

43 The Cellular Phone Task Force is dedicated to halting the expansion of wireless technology because it cannot be made safe. It provides education to the public concerning electromagnetic pollution (electrosmog); advocacy for an electromagnetically cleaner environment; and support for individuals disabled by radiation from wireless technology and other sources. See http://www.cellphonetaskforce.org/.

44 Rachel Carson's book, *Silent Spring* (1962), raised awareness of the growing harm being caused by the use of chemicals and pesticides on our crops and food.

45   I know that nutritional deficiencies can cause hearing loss also, and some people have fully regained their hearing using aldosterone supplements—thanks to the work of Dr Jonathan Wright, among others. People with age-related hearing loss may have only half of the aldosterone they need, says Dr Wright, in an interview with Suzanne Somers, in *Breakthrough* (2008). See also http://bit.ly/2ETP2VY.

46   For more details, See http://bit.ly/2ETCpul.

47   See p60 of the document: http://bit.ly/2FxIKg9.

48   See https://en.wikipedia.org/wiki/DBm.

49   See http://bit.ly/2ESGQpd.

50   See http://bit.ly/2ETo4xF.

51   Free download available here: https://olgasheean.com/heads-in-the-sand/.

52   Free download available here: http://bit.ly/2ET3AVW.

53   See http://bit.ly/2EPAlmN.

54   Free download available here: https://olgasheean.com/who-harm/.

55   See http://bit.ly/2EUVImE.

56   See https://olgasheean.com/who-emf/. You can add your name to the list, if you wish. More names are added daily, from people all over the world.

57   See http://bit.ly/2hlNEyK.

58   See http://wapo.st/2ig2Lfj.

59   See http://bit.ly/2isSXyb.

60   See http://bit.ly/2EQPDI3.

61   See http://bit.ly/2EPKikh.

62   See http://bit.ly/2ESeMCe.

63   See http://bit.ly/2EUW7Wc.

64   See http://bit.ly/2EO5Eyn.

65   See http://bit.ly/2gI34RW; on webpage, click on 'translate' for English version.

66   Other landmark rulings can be found here: http://bit.ly/2ESUubH.

67 See http://bit.ly/2EOqpKj.

68 See http://bit.ly/1CKLqQT and scroll down for the live-blood-analysis images and data.

69 See www.emf-portal.org.

70 *Evolve Your Brain* (2007) and *Breaking the Habit of Being Yourself* (2012).

71 For testimonials from those who have healed themselves using chi lel, see http://bit.ly/2FF3Bhk. For a healing meditation, see http://bit.ly/2Fcnb6L.

72 Why we are wired to connect, *Scientific American*, 22 October 2013, by Gareth Cook. See http://bit.ly/2ERMsjw.

73 Why loneliness hurts the heart. How this chronic form of stress can lead to heart disease. Ray Hainer, *Health*, 14 February 2012. See http://bit.ly/2ESffnY.

74 When people work together, they're literally on the same wavelength, brain waves show. Melissa Healy, *Los Angeles Times*, 28 April 2017. See http://lat.ms/2EToN1R.

75 Your smartphone is making you stupid, antisocial and unhealthy. So why can't you put it down? *The Globe and Mail*, 6 January 2018. See https://tgam.ca/2ESyZaU.

76 As per note 75.

77 See http://bit.ly/2EToYKz.

78 See http://bit.ly/2ESnKiW.

79 See http://bit.ly/29HnwgQ.

80 In *Psychology Today*. See http://bit.ly/1FYpfuP.

81 Is modern technology killing us? *Truthout*, op-ed, 19 September 2014. See http://bit.ly/2EPC6Ap.

82 See http://bit.ly/2EToYKz and http://resetyourchildsbrain.com.

83 How technical devices influence children's brains, 18 May 2015, *Psychology Today*. See http://bit.ly/1S0DphM.

84 See note 83.

85 When screens harm our children, *Tribune de Genève*, 26 August 2017. For original article in French, See http://bit.ly/2FtlrE7; for the English translation, see http://bit.ly/2ESIw1Z.

86   See http://bit.ly/2ERPiFb and http://bit.ly/2ER2v0M.

87   Personal communications. I spoke to Barrie on the phone in January 2018, and he confirmed the validity of these two accounts, adding that the first case was presented to British Parliament in 2005.

88   See minute 7.50: http://bit.ly/2ERPiFb.

89   See http://bit.ly/2DaxNSV.

90   See http://bit.ly/2EPCleN.

91   The Egoscue Method (also referred to as postural therapy) was devised to restore alignment by reintroducing motion that strengthens and re-engages temporarily dysfunctional supporting muscles and other musculoskeletal components. It's a natural way of addressing injury and chronic pain without resorting to toxic drugs or invasive surgery. See www.egoscue.com.

92   See http://bit.ly/2EQwohS.

93   For details of how the brain, mood, concentration and health are affected by using digital gadgets, causing mental illness and Internet Use Disorder (IUD) among millions of digital addicts, See http://bit.ly/2ET5ohG.

94   See http://dailym.ai/2ESIUNZ.

95   See http://bit.ly/2ETQKqm.

96   See http://bit.ly/2ESzOk0 (The biology of perception) and http://bit.ly/2EQR8pF (The biology of belief).

97   Another excellent resource for those wishing to re-wire their brains and upgrade their lives is the neural reprogramming work of Annie Hopper. See www.retrainingthebrain.com.

98   How Einstein revealed the universe's strange 'nonlocality'. George Musser, Scientific American, 1 November 2015. See http://bit.ly/2ER2YA4.

99   See http://bit.ly/2ETQXd8.

100 From Dr Joe Dispenza's Morning Meditation. See https://drjoedispenza.com.

101 Can our brain waves affect our physical reality? Peter Baksa, Huffington Post, 26 November 2011. See http://bit.ly/2ESJcV5.

102 The Quantum Doctor (2011), p59.

103 See http://bit.ly/2ETrnF5.

104 See https://drjoedispenza.com and https://masteringalchemy.com, respectively.

About the author

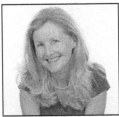

Olga Sheean is a writer, educator, relationship counsellor and empowerment coach specializing in human dynamics and quantum potential. An 'archaeologist of the mind', she is dedicated to excavating the deeper truth buried in every complex, amazing, powerful human being. Using her own unique framework for self-mastery, she helps people transform the negative subconscious programs that drive their circumstances, relationships, self-worth and success.

Olga has worked as a photojournalist for the World Wide Fund for Nature (WWF) International in Switzerland and as an editor for the United Nations in Geneva. A former magazine editor and health columnist, she is a prolific writer who has published over 300 articles in various magazines and regularly feeds her two blogs: *The O Zone—a place of positive e-missions* and *Beyond Belief—exposing the deeper truth.*

She is the author of four books:

- *Fit for Love: find your self and your perfect mate*
- *Gut Feelings—the inside story*
- *The Alphabet of Powerful Existence: an A–Z guide to well-being, wisdom and worthiness*
- *A Talk on the Wild Side—imaginary interviews with unlikely sources of wisdom*

In her downtime, she does kundalini yoga, plays 'silly Scrabble' (inventing new words), bounces on her 14-foot trampoline, enjoys reckless, rule-free table tennis, and reads voraciously.

Until further notice from the universe, she lives in British Columbia, Canada, with her husband, Lewis Evans.

For more info or to contact Olga, please see her empowerment website (https://olgasheean.com), where you can read about relationships and empowered, holistic living, access her blogs, purchase her books and recorded affirmations, download her free documents on electromagnetic radiation, and sign up for her newsletter. Her EMF website provides further details about this book, as well as a blog, additional resources and information about electromagnetic radiation: https://emfoff.com.

CPSIA information can be obtained
at www.ICGtesting.com
Printed in the USA
LVHW02s2339070818
586327LV00009B/338/P

9 781928 103103